ABAM 33 ?? / 'ET

HEALING BROKEN HURTS

GROWING THROUGH DIVORCE

REV. NELSON M. CHAMBERLIN

PUBLISHED BY FASTPENCIL

Published by FastPencil
3131 Bascom Ave.
Suite 150
Campbell CA 95008 USA
info@fastpencil.com
(408) 540-7571
(408) 540-7572 (Fax)
http://www.fastpencil.com

Dedicated to my wife (LaDonna Chamberlin) who co-anchored and counseled with me in each of the 44 Divorce Recovery Workshops we conducted over the years touching the lives of more than 800 hurting people
And to all those participants of our Workshops who contributed to our understanding of the trauma of divorce and who offered helpful suggestions that enhanced our program

ॐ

Acknowledgments

Lori Fisher —
(Placement Director at Indianapolis International Business College) who designed my book cover and guided me into the book publishing business

Audi Cathcart —
(Clinical Consultant with ProActive Medical Review) who advised me as to the content of this book

Monte Chamberlin —
(Founder and Owner of Cost Stewardship Company) who has been my advisor in all things financial

CONTENTS

1

A WAKE UP CALL

In 1975 I was assigned as minister of the Fishers United Methodist Church in Fishers, Indiana. My District Superintendent approached me with a deal I could hardly afford to turn down. He informed me that the Rev. Robert Schuller at the Crystal Cathedral Church in Garden Grove, California must be doing something right. He was conducting a Seminar for Successful Ministers and I was invited to attend with the idea of discovering some of the secrets of successful ministry. My Superintendent offered to help pay some of the expenses for that trip if I would in turn report to him what I had discovered.

I flew out to Los Angeles and attended the five-day seminar. I discovered many ideas I could utilize back in my church at Fishers. I was impressed first with his

Drive-In Worship Service. They had installed individual outdoor movie-type sound receivers for each car to be placed on their windows. Individuals from the church were there to welcome them and direct them to their places for worship. Their setting was picturesque and the quality of their presentation of worship was impressive.

I returned to Fishers and started the first Drive-In Worship in the Indianapolis Area. We had four loud speakers installed on the roof of our church building that could "blow" sound for five miles (if we wanted them to). We built an outdoor brick pulpit and lectern stand near the entry doors in the South Parking Lot, wired it for sound, and we were in business.

Our local Boy Scout Troop 109 was enlisted to help us in every service. They welcomed the Drive-In Worshippers, passed out bulletins and hymnals and collected them when the service was over.   They passed the offering plates through the congregated cars and delivered the gifts to our church treasurer when finished.

We pre-recorded the piano accompaniment for the hymns we sang and played them through the loudspeakers while the people sang in their cars. This service was appealing to many of our worshippers. Some were handicapped and could not get out of their cars to worship in our sanctuary. Others had physical problems like i and felt they would not be comfortable in a crowded sanctuary. There were some who had small children and they could bring them to the Drive-In Worship in their pajamas. We had worshippers who rode their horses to the services, and others who rode their bicycles ten miles to worship in the outdoors.

We had a great following in this early 8:30 a.m. service and had nearly 125 regular worshippers there (in addition to the regular services in the sanctuary). Our church grew exponentially in those days, and we soon had to add to our physical plant.

We upgraded our musical program and brought in nationally known vocalists (some of whom came from the Garden Grove Community Church, others from famous choirs like the Purdue University Glee Clubs).

But the thing that was most impressive to me about the Crystal Cathedral (and the thing that completely altered my ministry) was the Divorce Recovery Workshop that continued for a few days after the Successful Church Leadership was concluded. THAT WAS MY REAL WAKE-UP CALL!

The Rev. Jim Smoke was minister of Single Adults there at Garden Grove. He had 1200 single adults among their congregation. For several days I listened to him and these hurting people pour out their hearts, sat with them in restaurants hearing what it was like to have gone through a devastating divorce, and I was moved profoundly by that experience.

I came home to discover 82 single adults in our congregation. Basically as a congregation we were saying to them, "You are welcome here, but sit back over there in the corner and don't make much noise. We don't want to be bothered by you." I know why many churches won't deal with single adults in a meaningful way. Those congregations are filled with many people whose marriages are shaky and they see single-adults as "foot-loose and fancy-free," a threat to their weak marriages.

I did not want our church to be like that. So I said to my wife (LaDonna), "Honey, I think we are going to start a Divorce Workshop here." She looked at me with an incredulous look on her face and said, "How in the world are we going to do that? How will we know what to do?" I read over fifty books on divorce and single adult life. Finally I went to my Administrative Board and proposed that we be given permission to do this kind of ministry, and they agreed. (Not fully understanding the need for this), but since they were used to me starting new "weird" things by now, they approved what was to be the changing event in my life.

My wife and I conducted 44 Divorce Recovery Workshops ministering to over 800 people up to and past our retirement. It has been the absolutely most rewarding experience we have had in all of our ministry! Others have taken cues from our experiences and have designed Divorce Recovery Workshops of their own. One of my associates at Fishers went from here to the largest United Methodist Church in the South Conference and built a large single adult fellowship that touched many people.

Because of that WAKE UP CALL, I am now sharing some insights in this book that I hope will inspire other individuals and congregations to reach out and touch their friends whose lives have been broken and need help.

2

GETTING STARTED

Of all the more than 50 books I read on the subject of marriage and divorce, Jim Smoke's book "Growing Through Divorce" was the most influential to me. I borrowed heavily from his book to organize our program. You may find it helpful as well.

To begin ... we discovered that the place for meeting was better suited outside of the church building. Some participants may be reluctant to set feet inside a church. We conducted our workshops in a comfortable setting of sofas, chairs, tables, and a fire place in our own home (basement Great Room). We had a person ready at the front door to greet them and direct them to the place where we were meeting. We had a place to put their coats (on our pool table) where they could readily identify them when they were leaving. We noted where the restroom facilities could be located.

We served refreshments each night toward the end of the session when participants were encouraged to remain and share their thoughts and concerns with each other and with us. We promised that we would not conclude any session until the last person was ready to leave.

Paper plates, paper cups, paper napkins and plastic silverware were made available. A good supply of Kleenex was always available because tears tended to flow occasionally.

We charged a minimum fee ($30-$35) for the entire seven sessions, and offered scholarships for those who could not afford the fee. Once money is invested participants are more likely to attend each session, and we emphasize how vital this is because our workshops build upon each of the previous sessions. They were advised that if they were going to be unable to attend any session, we would provide them with a tape recording of that session so that they would not fall too far behind the other participants in this program. That recording would include only the input from the leaders but would exclude all the comments by the people attending.

OUR SCHEDULE

Session One — "Does Anyone Know Or Care How I Feel?"

Session Two — "How To Cope With Your Ex-Spouse"

Session Three — "Forgiveness ... Finding A New Start In Life"

Session Four — "How To Assume Responsibility ... For Yourself, Your Children, and Your Future"

Session Five — " What Do I Do With All That Money I Don't Have Anymore?"

Session Six — " Hey, God! What Do I Do About Sex?"

Session Seven — " To Live and Love Again"

We note from the beginning: In consideration of all participants, things that are revealed in confidence here among us are agreed to remain confidential. We want to develop a sense of mutual trust and confidence in this group. Your understanding and agreement is essential to the success of this workshop.

We began each session at 7:15 P.M. with Coffee and an Informal Get-Together.

At 7:25 P.M. we had what we called SHOW-AND-TELL-TIME which offered participants the opportunity to report on the progress they had made toward the goals they had set for themselves the previous week. Those who set goals and achieved some progress usually were anxious to share where they had come from. Those who failed to set goals for themselves or were unable to see much personal progress were usually reluctant to participate in this discussion. We emphasized strongly the importance of setting personal goals for themselves each week.

At 7:35 P.M. we delivered what was called THE KEY-NOTE ADDRESS. In subsequent chapters you will discover the text of some of those Keynote Addresses.

At 8:00 P.M. we opened the class for GROUP DISCUSSIONS AND EXERCISES led by my wife (LaDonna). A list of questions was offered each evening in which we encouraged the class to respond and discuss. Some of those will be seen in later chapters.

At 8:45 P.M. we had what was termed THE POST-GAME SHOW in which participants were encouraged to get separated with other participants and share their personal lives with each other. We discovered that as time went on many of them would arrange to meet with other classmates at restaurants during the week to share more and develop close friendships. We made ourselves available during the Post-Game Show to counsel individually with those who felt the need to do so, and we remained until the last person was gone.

3

SESSION ONE — "DOES ANYONE KNOW OR CARE HOW I FEEL?"

Many people who suffer the hurt of divorce feel that no one ever hurt as badly as they do. They wonder if anybody knows or cares how much the trauma of divorce brings them pain. So my first Key-Note address was this:

Does anyone know or care how I feel?

That question is intended to be a 'grabber.' It is designed to capture your attention and gain your ear. BUT IT IS A SERIOUS QUESTION because I know that many of you are here this evening experiencing some very deep and wrenching emotions. Some of you are probably thinking, 'NOBODY ELSE EVER HAD IT AS BAD AS I HAVE IT. NOBODY EVER FELT LIKE

I FEEL RIGHT NOW. NOBODY COULD EVER
BEGIN TO UNDERSTAND WHAT I AM GOING
THROUGH!'

And if you care to stretch that a little farther, you
might even push it to the point where you are saying (or
thinking), 'WHAT CAN THAT HAPPILY MARRIED
MAN UNDERSTAND OR KNOW ABOUT LIFE
THAT WOULD GIVE HIM THE AUDACITY TO
GET   UP   THERE   AND   TALK   TO   ME
ABOUT   **GROWING   THROUGH   DIVORCE?**'
That's all right. See ... I already know how some of you
feel ... and that should be a comfort to you and not a
threat.

One of my good friends is a Catholic priest. He told
me that once he was asked how he could stand up in
front of his parishioners and give them advice about
family-planning, birth control, and raising children when
he had never had any first-hand experience in any of
those areas. (That was a good question ... don't you
think!) But he had a better answer. He responded,
'DOES A VETERINARIAN HAVE TO BE A HORSE
TO TREAT A SICK ANIMAL?'

The truth of the matter is that people can and do care
how you feel if they find it in their hearts to take the time
to listen. I first awoke to what it is like to be single and
divorced when I attended a seminar at Bob Schuller's
Garden Grove Community Church in Garden Grove,

California. I was sent there by my District Superintendent with the instructions, "He certainly is doing
some things right. Go out there and find out what it is,
report back to me and I will help you out with your
expenses." I attended the Successful Church Leaders
Conference for several days.

Then I learned that immediately upon the heels of this
conference was to follow a conference on Single Adult
Ministries. Jim Smoke was the minister of Single Adult
Ministries in that church. More than 1200 people were
single adult members of that congregation. Since I had
spent all that money to get out there, I decided to stay a
few days more and take in this conference as well. For
three days I listened to broken-hearted, beautiful, sensi-
tive people as they poured out their bleeding guts about
how it feels to go through the trauma of divorce. Those
three days radically changed my life and my ministry.

I came home to talk in depth with some of my best
friends ... a minister, a lawyer, a house wife, an office
worker, a business man ... all of whom had gone
through the trauma of divorce. I discovered 82 single
adults in my congregation at that time. And we as a congregation were saying (in essence), "This is a family
church and you are welcome here. But just sit back over
there in the corner and don't make a whole lot of noise."

One of my single adult friends was a lawyer who had
seen three marriages explode in his face. He is a good

United Methodist who enjoys an occasional drink in some of the local pubs, so I figured he would be an excellent guide to some of the singles bars in the area. I decided I would let him take me bar-hopping one night just so that I might sit down over a coke and talk with some of those lonely people to discover what life was like as they were now experiencing it. The night before we were scheduled to go together, my friend was taken to I.U. Med Center for back surgery, and my bar-hopping days came to an abrupt end before they ever got started. I don't know if the Lord was trying to tell me something important in that or not. I did not get to go!

But I have tried my dead level best to understand what people in your shoes are experiencing. I have done considerable research making this the new focus of my specialty in ministry. My wife and I have worked with several hundred people just like you who were struggling through divorce. And even though I have been married to this neat lady here for more than 50 years, WE HAVE NEVER ONCE THOUGHT ABOUT DIVORCE ... *(LENGTHY PAUSE WAITING FOR THEIR NEGATIVE REACTION)* ... NEVER ONCE THOUGHT ABOUT DIVORCING EACH OTHER ...**MURDER EIGHT TIMES, BUT NEVER DIVORCE!** (They finally smile and we go on.)

We come this evening with a wealth of experience because other good people just like you have given us the privilege of walking down the private corridors of their own minds and hearts, and they have shared with us how it feels to be single and hurting.

So let me share with you what I see as the purpose and goal of our being here together tonight and for the next six weeks. If any of you are here expecting to get a good pistol-whipping with the Bible, I am afraid you may go away disappointed. If any of you need to have an over-worked sense of guilt reinforced in you, you will probably have to look elsewhere.

LaDonna and I would like to share with you some information we believe will be helpful in making it possible for you to **GROW** THROUGH DIVORCE rather than simply to **GO** THROUGH DIVORCE. In the process of our sharing with you, we hope you will share with us because we learn from you as well as sharing what we have learned from others.

I see the purpose of this workshop as DEVEL-OPING **A SUPPORTIVE FELLOWSHIP** that will meet some of the relational needs of your life. THE EMPHASIS IS GOING TO BE ON SUPPORT! You have already suffered more than you need to in the con-demnation and judgment of others. Sometimes church people are like that. I know why ... YOU ARE A THREAT TO THEM. THEY ARE SITTING THERE WITH SHAKY MARRIAGES OF THEIR OWN, AND HERE YOU COME FOOT-LOOSE AND FANCY-

FREE, and they can't stand that! So they push you over in an insignificant corner somewhere and at best ignore you ... or worst, they dump unneeded and unsolicited loads of guilt and condemnation on you.

You don't need any more of that, so we are going to concentrate on offering you a SUPPORTIVE FELLOW-SHIP. When this workshop is concluded, I can already guarantee that you are going to single out (no pun intended) others in this group whom you will be tele-phoning every once in awhile when you need support on a down day ... and some of these people may become your life-long friends. You need supportive friendships and we intend to make some of those possible for you.

Secondly, we want to build for you **A SOCIAL FEL-LOWSHIP** as well. No, my friends ... we are not in the match-making business. I suspect that none of you are ready for that anyway! But we can and will provide a place where wholesome friendships may become estab-lished and developed.

Thirdly, we want to build a **SPIRITUAL FELLOW-SHIP** that can help you deal with the problems of your emotions, your deepest feelings, your wounded spirits. What religious background you come from (if any) is of no vital concern to us. We have no intention of using this workshop to increase the number of members in our church. Believe me now ... this workshop is for you and our sole motivation is the hope of seeing you grow through divorce.

Now let me share with you some of the things we have learned about the trauma and heartbreak of divorce.

Whenever you lose something in which you invested a significant piece of yourself, you are going to go through the process of grief described by Elisabeth Kubler Ross i ner book   ... SHOCK, DENIAL, ANGER, GUILT, BARGAINING WITH GOD, HOPE, and finally ACCEPTANCE.

STAGE ONE

The first, almost universal emotion we experience in a broken relationship is SHOCK. "OH, DEAR GOD ... I KNOW THIS HAPPENS TO OTHER PEOPLE, BUT I NEVER THOUGHT IT WOULD HAPPEN TO ME." And yet here it is ... and it is happening to you. Divorce until this moment is only a statistic ... it happens in 41% of all first-time marriages, 59% of all second marriages, 83% of all third-time marriages. And 50% of the first time marriages being performed today are presumably destined for divorce. "Oh God ... it can't happen to me!" But it did! And that for many people spells shock!

What does shock do to us? Shock is a God-given reaction that protects us when the hurt we experience is too great to bear. Bang your head in an automobile accident, and if the injury is severe enough you go into shock where you are unaware of what is happening to you. Take a blow to the heart, a heartbreak, and if it is bad enough you may lose touch with reality. Some people retreat within themselves and block out all thoughts of what is happening to them. They deny it mentally. They refuse to talk about it with anyone. They withdraw from friends and social contacts. They move. They change jobs. And what they are doing basically is running away from the issue. "IF I JUST DON'T THINK ABOUT IT OR TALK ABOUT IT, IT MIGHT GO AWAY!" UNNGGHH, UNNGGHH!!! That is just so much hogwash.

Those confused inner feelings may run the gamut all the way from personal feelings of guilt for ever letting a thing like this happen to a sense of utter failure, or even the transference of those feelings to a totally different person.

NOW HOW DO WE GET UNSTUCK FROM THIS PARALYZING EMOTIONAL EXPERIENCE?

Growing through divorce begins with the admission that this really is happening to me ... because you will never adequately and honestly deal with the situation unless you can first admit that the situation exists. One who had gone through a large number of divorces was fond of telling her friends that she was merely "in between relationships." That is not honestly dealing with the situation.

When you face up to the situation, you may go through feelings of ANGER, BITTERNESS, LONELI-NESS, GUILT, FEAR, EMPTINESS, WEAKNESS, MOURNING, and hopefully you may eventually experience feelings of RELIEF, HOPE, JOY! We will talk about those feelings later.

One of the ways of prolonging the shock stage is to desparately and unrealistically cling to HOPE. I hear some saying, "There is still an outside chance that we might get back together." Or "I know he has not been good for me, but maybe if I tried harder ... maybe if I give him one more chance he might change."

WHERE DID WE EVER GET THE IDEA THAT MARRIAGE WAS INTENDED TO BE REFORM SCHOOL? We take people where they are, for whatever they are when we marry them. Jim Smoke writes in his book Growing Through Divorce ... "Getting married is like buying a phonograph record: You buy it for what's on one side but you have to take the flip side too." Then he adds "Getting divorced is like getting the hole in the record." WE DON'T MARRY PROJECTS ... WE MARRY PEOPLE!

People with unrealistic hopes come to the marriage counselor with ideas that he can do something that they cannot do for themselves. They come to their minister with the hope that he is some kind of miracle worker. They pray to God hoping that the fatal hurts they have inflicted on one another can be healed. Sometimes God does not respond affirmatively to that sort of false hope. You had better realize that sometimes God answers your prayers with the word "NO" instead of "YES." That too is an answer to your prayer.

Now let me offer several questions that will help you sort out false hope from reality.

1. DO BOTH PARTIES WANT THE MARRIAGE TO SUCCEED?

If both parties really want a shaky marriage to succeed, there is a high degree of realistic hope that the marriage can succeed providing they accept professional help. If one does not want the marriage to succeed, then it does not matter how strongly the other person wants it. IT TAKES TWO TO TANGO, and if there are not two people who are agreed that their marriage succeed, you would best just forget it. You have no other choice. That may not be the message you hoped to receive tonight, but that is the realistic truth and you would do well to accept it.

2. WILL BOTH PARTIES ACCEPT PROFESSIONAL HELP IN RECONCILIATION FOR AS LONG AS IS NECESSARY?

Counselors simply cannot work ONE-PARTY MIRACLES. You cannot undo in five minutes what it took fifteen years of wanton havoc to bring about. And you can't do it solo. To believe anything else is unrealistic.

3. HAS A THIRD PARTY BECOME INVOLVED WITH EITHER MATE?

Experience proves that third-party involvements tend to bring marriages to an end. Some partners will wait, forgive, endure and try to forget (though I doubt they will ever completely forget ... for how can you turn your memory on and off at will?). You have to remember what you are trying to forget in order to forget it.

There are a few exceptions to that rule, but the odds are greatly against you if you are hoping to make a HAPPY DUET out of an UNHAPPY TRIANGLE. It just is not that easy. It just doesn't work that often.

4. WHAT HAVE YOU LEARNED FROM YOUR PAST EXPERIENCES THAT WILL SHED LIGHT ON YOUR PRESENT SITUATION?

Hopefully, you will not have to marry as often as Zsa-Zsa Gabor or Elizabeth Taylor or Mickey Rooney to learn from experience. Many marriages contain elements that were out of control long before the marriage became a reality. But people still insist on gambling their lives and their well-being on the unrealistic hope that things will be different next time rather than facing reality.

You would do well to learn from the past. Discover the garbage you brought out of that previous relationship and deal with that garbage before you ever allow yourself to enter into another marriage relationship.

Otherwise you will be destined to live that tragedy all over again.

You see, it isn't really second or third marriages that are bad! It is carrying the same old garbage into those marriages that dooms them. So deal with the junk in your life. Get rid of it and give yourself a real chance at success next time around. We are going to help you deal with that very thing over the next several weeks.

STAGE TWO

As the shock of divorce begins to wear off, a process of ADJUSTMENT begins to take place. Shock means facing the facts of divorce. Adjustment means doing something about those facts. And this is an excellent place to GIVE A DEAD RELATIONSHIP A GOOD PROPER BURIAL. Mourn it if you will. Hurt if you choose to. Cry if it feels good. But don't be satisfied to swim in a sea of self-pity for the rest of your life.

Feeling sorry for yourself is not totally escapable, but I would like to suggest that it should be limited to a five second experience about once every other week! Is what you are looking for only a warehouse full of "I'm so sorry's" from your friends? Self-pity can be so self-defeating, so depressing, and that is why it is not good for you. you are the one that counts now. If you refuse to look out for yourself, who do you think is going to do it for you? Unnnggghhhuhhh! I think you got that one right!

STAGE THREE

This is the stage I covet for every one of you ... THE GROWTH STAGE. Jim Smoke in his book *Growing Through Divorce* says there are eight steps to growing through divorce.

1. REALIZE THAT TIME IS A HEALER and you must WALK THROUGH THAT PROCESS ONE DAY AT A TIME.

2. COME TO GRIPS WITH YOURSELF. YOU CANNOT DENY YOUR EXISTENCE NO MATTER HOW FRUSTRATED, LONELY, GUILTY, ANGRY, OR DESPARATE YOU MAY FEEL ON THE INSIDE.

3. SET ASIDE TIME FOR REFLECTION, MEDI-TATION, READING, THINKING AND PERSONAL GROWTH. Many situations you may never be able to change, but you can change yourself anytime you really want to.

4. GET TOGETHER WITH HEALTHY PEOPLE WHO ARE STRUGGLING BUT GROWING. There is only minimal comfort in hearing other peoples' divorce stories while you are going through divorce. At first it may help, but soon it becomes boring. Healthy people are those who let the past die and who live and grow in the present.

5. SEEK PROFESSIONAL COUNSELING OR THERAPY IF YOU NEED IT. Asking for help is a sign of strength ... not a sign of weakness.

6. ACCEPT THE FACT THAT YOUR ARE
DIVORCED (OR IN THE PROCESS OF BEING
DIVORCED) AND YOU ARE NOW SINGLE.   It
ought not to hurt too badly to say it. So repeat after me:
"I AM SINGLE ... AND I'M OK!"

7. PUT THE PAST IN THE PAST WHERE IT
BELONGS AND BEGIN TO LIVE IN THE
PRESENT.

8. COMMIT YOUR NEW WAY TO GOD. BEGIN
NEW THINGS, AND SEEK THE HELP AND RELA-
TIONSHIPS YOU NEED TO BEGIN ANEW.

I'm going to back off now and let my co-partner lead
you in the Discussion Exercise.

The first session Discussion was centered around
some of the feelings that were most prevalent in their
lives. LaDonna encouraged them by saying, "We can
learn a lot from you, and others will learn a lot too if you
will take the courage to share. Tell us what you are
feeling and what you are struggling with."

Several were able to be open and share while other
were reluctant and hesitant to share their feelings. One
fellow could do nothing but cry the whole first session.
Another confessed he was devastated that he found his
closest friend in bed with his wife when he came home
early one afternoon.

Another explained that the feeling he was experiencing was abject loneliness. One of the dear ladies who seemed at the time to have all the words but none of the "music" responded immediately, "I have discovered that since I have Jesus in my heart, I never have to feel lonely" ... to which he responded immediately "Bovine Droppings!" (Well, that is not exactly how he put it. "BULL S*#T" is what he actually said, and the class burst out in laughter and acceptance of what he was feeling and saying.)

The purpose and goal of that first session was to help them realize that there are many feelings that are prevalent in their situation and it is all right to have those feelings. How we manage those feelings is the more important thing, and that is the theme for the second session.

4

SESSION TWO — "HOW TO COPE WITH YOUR EX-SPOUSE"

The second session should really be titled *"How To Cope With YOUR FEELINGS About Your Ex-Spouse"* (because it continues with the theme about feelings ... how to handle them in dealing with your ex-spouse).

Again we began with coffee and the informal get-together at 7:15 P.M. You can measure the enthusiasm for the course among the participants by noting who comes early (before the announced starting time of 7:30 P.M.).

At 7:25 P.M. we had our first official SHOW AND TELL TIME. We inquired:

1. Did you select a personal goal for the past week?

2. What progress did you make toward that goal?

3. How do you feel about this class for far?

That last question was a "loaded" question. It was designed to show us (and them) about the difficulties of really expressing feelings. People who responded about what they liked or did not like were not getting deep into their inner feelings. People who said they were SAD, SCARED, ANGRY, GUILTY, HOPEFUL, RELIEVED were people who were getting into their real feelings. That is how they will be able to cope with their ex-spouse and their feelings toward them.

We passed out a sheet called **S.M.A.R.T. GOALS.** It informed them —

At the end of each session we encourage participants to take a few moments reflect in silence upon what they have heard that evening, and then to establish for themselves at least one S.M.A.R.T. goal they will seek to achieve during the coming week.

S.M.A.R.T. goals are

Specific Goals ... It is not enough to promise yourself "I will become a better person   this week." That is not specific enough. The goal needs to be more like "I will talk   with my spouse on the phone this week and not allow myself to get carried away in anger." Or "I will take an honest look at my finances and formulate a plan for getting things under control."

Measurable Goals ... It is essential that goals can be measured so that one may   know when that goal has been achieved. Perhaps your goal might be to reach out to some of your friends for help. "I will talk to three of my best friends ... Mary, Suzie and John ... to tell them about what I am doing to get my life back in order." When you measure up to the requirements of that goal, that is a goal being accomplished ... but not until!

Achievable Goals ... Goals must be achievable. "I will get ahold of $1,000,000 this week" may not be an achievable goal (unless you know something the rest of us do not know). But "I will make at least three appointments for interviews for a new job" may be more achievable.

Realistic Goals ... "I will never allow that person to speak to my children again, even if I have to shoot him to prevent it." S.M.A.R.T. goals must be reasonable and rational.

Timely Goals ... A scheduled deadline can be helpful in enabling you to achieve your S.M.A.R.T. goals. If there is no time-line for the completion of your goal, you may allow yourself to dawdle forever without getting the job done. "I will do this by no later than 5:00 o'clock next Tuesday so that I can report to the DRW (Divorce Recovery Workshop)." That would be a timely goal.

Bob Schuller is fond of saying, "If you fail to plan, then you plan to fail." Goal-setting   is an essential element in GROWING through divorce. JUST DO IT!

My KEYNOTE ADDRESS for this evening was:

People who are committed to growth are not hung up in the past, nor are they frozen into inaction by fears about the future. People who are growing through divorce are interested in making their lives meaningful in the HERE AND NOW!

But one of the greatest struggles that must be faced in divorce is the struggle of LETTING GO of the many things that were a part of the marriage experience. One of the last vestiges to go in a broken marriage is the comfort and security of having a PHYSICAL PRESENCE around you to whom you can speak, to whom you can turn when you are in difficulty, and to whom you can move when the pangs of loneliness are about to do you in.

Our feelings (of which we spoke in considerable depth last week) are such complicating factors in achieving Growth THROUGH divorce. Those feeling can go so rapidly from love ... to hate ... to revenge. And those feelings may not stand pat in one place for long. They can go from love to hate to revenge and back to love again in the short space of a few seconds. Some keep engaging in that battle for many long years without ever coming out the victor.

So the question tonight is 'HOW DO I DEAL WITH MY EX-SPOUSE?' But it may go deeper than that! 'HOW DO I DEAL WITH **MY FEELINGS** ABOUT MY EX-SPOUSE?'

Dr. Robert S. Weiss in his book *Marital Separation* says "Separation is an *incident* in the relationship. It is a critically important incident, to be sure: an incident that ushers in fundamental changes in the relationship. **BUT IT IS NOT THE ENDING.**"

When the Judge says "Divorce granted" or "Dissolution allowed," that does not mean that your relationship is totally and irrevocably terminated. It simply means you don't have to live together anymore as husband and wife. There are a thousand and one times when you will have to deal with each other ... when you may have to face each other ...when the battle is renewed or at least attempted to be renewed through the children ... when the financial situation is cause for concern and consultation.

Divorce is not the end of a relationship. It is only the official recognition of the state and society that the relationship from this time forward will be on DIFFERENT GROUNDS and under DIFFERENT GROUND RULES. And ohhh ... how the emotions can complicated this new relationship!

Jim Smoke says there are SEVEN BASIC CAUSES OF DIVORCE THAT SEEM TO APPEAR WITH THE MOST FREQUENCY. They are:

1. THE VICTIM DIVORCE. This is where one partner leaves the home for another person ... his secretary ... her old boyfriend, or whatever. It matters not who ... THE RESULTS ARE ALL THE SAME. ONE PERSON WANTS THE DIVORCE WHILE THE OTHER PERSON DOES NOT. The mate left behind may suffer feelings of rejection, abandonment, worthlessness, despair, and even guilt that can soon turn into ANGER and REVENGE (very messy emotions, I might add). HOSTILITY toward the ex-spouse is **2. THE PROBLEM DIVORCE.** This is a divorce predicated upon a problem the other person had. Some of these problems may include alcohol, drugs, gambling, money management, sexual inabilities, psychological shortcomings, gnawing physical problems ... (none of which were ever resolved). Some people bring their problems into the marriage with them while others are created within and because of the marriage itself. Some people bargain for the problems when they contract the marriage.

Dr. Eric Byrne in his book *"Games People Play"* gives us the insight that often the person who marries an active alcoholic is asking for the punishment that God or the rest of society seems unwilling to give her because she is such a bad person and actually deserves to be punished. She says to herself, "I will marry that loser, and then I may get the punishment I deserve."

THAT IS SICK ... IT IS SAD ... BUT IT IS TRUE! People who are victims of Problem Divorces experience feelings that run all the way from SYMPATHY for the ex-mate to the REGRET that so many years were wasted on that kind of existence. The person with the problem is most likely to feel ABANDONMENT. You have heard of the expression "CO-DEPENDENCY." Well, you are looking at it right there.

I've got to add one more observation here. There are some kind and beautiful people who seemingly have a MESSIAH COMPLEX. They see a needy person and think they can rescue them ... save them. Preacher's kids are especially vulnerable to this kind of relationship.

They marry "PROJECTS" without realizing how doomed such a relationship can be. Far too often these marriages end in disaster with the same feelings predominant as described previously in the Problem Divorce.

3. THE LITTLE GIRL/LITTLE BOY DIVORCE. This divorce is brought about when one mate or the other decides they do not want the responsibilities of being husband or wife, father or mother any longer. They decide they want to spend their time with the "boys" or the "girls" and play with the kind of toys they played with before their marriage. The only difference seems to be the price of the toys! We see a lot of this in

the Hollywood Jet Set and the Playboy's Club mentality. PERSONAL IMMATURITY and the LACK OF LEARNING TO ACCEPT RESPONSIBILITY bring on this kind of divorce. Feelings here for the one left behind are centered in unbelievable REJECTION while the offender goes along feeling little or nothing at all except the joy of doing something different.

4. THE "I WAS CONNED" DIVORCE. In simplest terms this means that one mate did not get what he or she was counting on when they entered into the marriage. It happens all too often in whirlwind romances where the couple scarcely has time to get to know each other. But it happens also when one person finds it impossible to be honest with the other ... hence the disillusionment ... hence the divorce. This kind of divorce usually leads toward a DEFENSIVENESS toward the ex-spouse and a GENERAL DISTRUST OF THE OPPOSITE SEX. That continued sort of reaction does not make for very good prospects of a successful marriage to another.

5. THE SHOTGUN WEDDING. Most of us have heard of "shotgun" weddings before ... you know, where the guests throw puffed rice instead of the usual kind. These weddings are usually initiated by the fact that the bride-to-be is pregnant. In my experience in pre-marital counseling, I have run into lots of young people who think I have never studied the principles of higher math-

ematics. But I do know how to add 5+4, 6+3, 7+2, and so on. Because a pregnancy is involved, in many cases the bride feels pressured by family and friends and community to marry the father of the child-to-be, and the boy feels pressured by the girl to marry her.

Fathers of the bride don't escort the couple to the altar of the church with a shotgun in hand, but the pressure is still often there. When the rare couple informs me that the reason they want to get married is 'BECAUSE WE HAVE TO,' my first question is 'WHO SAYS SO? WHO SAYS YOU HAVE TO GET MARRIED?'

Where there is no genuine (1)LOVE, (2) GENUINE TRUST, (3)GENUINE COMMUNICATION, (4)GENUINE COMPATIBILITY OR MUTUALITY, there is little chance of a marriage succeeding, and even the pressure of the shotgun cannot hold such an ill-advised union together. The predominant feeling in such a breakup is GUILT.

6. THE MENOPAUSE DIVORCE. We used to think that only women go through menopause, but now we know differently. We know that men also go through some kind of change in life similar to women in menopause. I both sexes, dramatic changes in personality and behavior can cause one mate or the other to leave the marriage. My own personal observation is that especially as persons in their forties begin to realize that they are losing their youth and vigor, they become desperate and sometimes covenant with themselves, "IF I COULD JUST FIND SOMEONE WHO WOULD LOVE ME (what horrible crimes we do to the word "love"), THEN MAYBE I COULD PROVE TO MYSELF I AM NOT OVER THE HILL YET."

And so in an effort to deny their mortality and their natural aging process, and to boost their deflated egos in an extra-marital affair, the menopause divorce occurs. Attitudes toward the ex-spouse after this kind of divorce are centered in SURPRISE, COMPLETE LACK OF UNDERSTANDING, and a GENERAL CONFUSION as to what happened and why. Because this often occurs after many years of marriage, a DEEP HURT and BIT-TERNESS is coupled with a feeling of BETRAYAL AND ABANDONMENT.

7. **THE NO-FAULT DIVORCE.** Several years ago, parties who were applying for divorce where required to make charges against each other in the courts. Charges and counter-charges made for a lively scene, and specta-tors relished the unfolding of the drama like they now can get in their daily soap-operas on television. Some-body had to be made out the villain.

Today the scene in Divorceland USA is changed. Nobody has to be at fault. The two simply must declare, "Sorry, your Honor, but both of us have tried and it just isn't going to work for either of us." No dirty linen to hang out on the lines ... no rancorous bitterness accompanying the proceedings ... just a simple "We want out" and they can go their separate ways. There are things that could be said on both sides of this issue, but I am not going to take the time to debate this tonight ... except to say I DON'T THINK TOO EASY DIVORCE IS THE PROBLEM. I THINK TOO EASY MARRIAGE IS THE CULPRIT!

In the NO-FAULT DIVORCE, feelings are usually very neutral. They simply acknowledge their marriage did not work out, wish each other better luck next time, and go their separate ways. **HEAR ME NOW ... NO NEED TO FIX THE BLAME ANYMORE ... JUST FIX THE PROBLEM!**

It is vitally important for you to realize in which category (or categories) of divorce you fall. And it is easiest to determine that by identifying the feelings that were strongest in your mind when you went through divorce.

That should be a clue for you to determine the real cause of your divorce.

While the hurt is most intense while the wounds of the divorce are still fresh, as time passes and new interests and relationships are formed, the conflict level will subside. BUT THAT CAN NEVER HAPPEN AS LONG AS YOU LIVE IN THE PAST ... NURSING THOSE HURTS, NURSING THE GUILT, OR NURSING THE LONELINESS THAT IS SO MUCH

A PART OF THOSE EARLY DAYS AFTER DIVORCE. How can you accept the present or plan for the future if you are longing for or living in the past?

The hurts that you have experienced through divorce may remain for a time, but at least the aggravation level will go down in time if you give it a chance. Growth in dealing with an ex-spouse takes place when your feelings of hostility, hatred and revenge mellow first to feelings of guilt and feeling sorry for yourself, and finally they mellow to acceptance. This process of time and working through your feelings may take a long time. There is no instant cure (though many search for it in a quick marriage). Beware ... hurt feelings take time to heal.

Next we passed out a sheet (**Pertinent Points**) recounting the seven basic causes of divorce and La Donna led them in a discussion of this. Then she introduced **GROWTH GUIDELINES** which included the following:

1. Take the detachment one day at a time.
2. Try to make the break as clean as possible.
3. Quit accepting responsibility for the ex-spouse.
4. Do not let your children intimidate you.
5. Do not get trapped in your "child" state.

"Growth in divorce is treating an ex-spouse as an adult. It is not seeking reprisal and vindication even if you feel deserving of it. Negative and childish treatment of an ex-spouse is immature and a constant drain on your emotional

level. Warring people are in a constant state of battle tension. Little positive growth is attained until the fight is declared over. In your dealing with your ex-spouse, tell them that your part of the war is over! If they continue to fight, let it be their problem and do not continue to supply them with ammunition."

I then offered four items that dealt with handling emotions with your ex-spouse. The first was **THE PHYSIOLOGY OF ANGER.**

There's nothing wrong with anger. Anger is a gift of God. The Bible tells us it is all right to be angry. "Be angry and sin not," it tells us. Jesus was a person totally capable of great anger. So it is not wrong to be angry. But what we do with anger can sometimes be harmful. So anger has to be used in wholesome and productive ways.

Anger is a gift of God that prepares us for fight or flight. It is part of the nature ingrained in us since the beginning of the animal kingdom. Anger prepares us or our animal friends to run or else that stick it out and battle when we are in danger.

Anger turns on the adrenaline in our systems so that we have more energy to run or fight.

Anger turns on the clotting mechanism in our blood so that if we are wounded we may not be so susceptible of bleeding to death.

Anger turns off the blood supply to our stomach, since the blood may have more important things to do at the moment rather than merely digesting food.

Anger increases the blood pressure so that the flow of blood in our system is at a sufficiently higher level so that we can do what the situation demands of us

Anger does many things for us physically so that we can run or fight. But if we do neither ... if we turn that anger upon ourselves ... If we stuff it and do not use it for its intended use, then those very things done for us in our bodies began to work against us. Stomach aches, blood clots, hypertension, dissipation of energy... These aren't just a few of the things that unresolved anger can bring us.

Next I gave an example of **HARNESSING THE ENERGY OF ANGER.**

Sandy was a redhead and Sandy was angry. She had a reason to be. After working so hard to accumulate what she and her husband had been able to do, her husband abandoned her... divorced her. He and his three lawyers took advantage of her and worked her over to the tune of more than $300,000 in legal fees and other schemes. They did little or nothing for her in performing their services ... and left her broken financially as well as emotionally.

Sandy expressed her anger quite vociferously in our Divorce Recovery Workshop ... and I encourage her to do that. But finally we came to the point where I had to ask her, "All right, Sandy... What are you going to do with that anger? How are you going to channel it into something productive? What do you plan to do with that anger?" She did not know but she promised she would think about it.

The next week Sandy came to Divorce Recovery Workshop a new person. She was radiant with happiness. She had found a purpose in living. "I know what I am going to do with my anger," she told us. "I am going to start a lawyer-referral program for women like myself who are going through divorce. I am going to get a list of all the good lawyers, and I am going to get a list of the bad lawyers they need to be aware of. And I am going to make a living sharing with other women what I've learned the hard way."

Sandy is a longtime friend of ours who lives in Chesterfield, Indiana. Even after 15 years she occasionally stops by our house or writes to us to tell us what is happening in her life. I don't know if ever she ever got back her $300,000, but I do know that she got back something far more important than that. She got control over her life. She found something worth living for. She found something to do with our anger. She channeled the energy that was literally eating her alive, put it to a useful purpose, and saved her life and health in the process.

So what are you going to do with your anger? Are you going to let it eat you up or are you going to find a way to do something constructive with it?

I have learned a great deal from the writings of the American psychotherapist and psychologist Albert Ellis and one of his compatriots Dr. Jeffrey Barnes dealing with the psychological approach called Rational Emotive Therapy. I shared this with the group.

RATIONAL EMOTIVE THERAPY (R.E.T.)

I took a course at the University of Indianapolis taught by Dr. Jeffery Barnes, a practicing psychiatrist at the Indiana University Medical Center. In the course of his presentation he taught us about a field of psychiatry called "Rational Emotive Therapy." RET advocates assert that *THERE IS NO DIRECT RELATIONSHIP BETWEEN WHAT HAPPENS TO US AND HOW WE FEEL ABOUT IT.* That of course was hard for me to comprehend or accept at first.

Dr. Barnes clarified the RET principle with this illustration. He pointed at me and said, "Chamberlin ... if somebody walked into this classroom right now, went over to where you are sitting, and put a gun to your head, what would you be feeling?" "Scared to death!" I replied. "Good," he responded — Probably a very appropriate response for that event."

Then he asked, "Would everybody feel that same fear that you felt?" "Sure they would," I answered confidently. "Oh no, they would not," he countered. "Oh yes, they would," I asserted again.

"Well now, what if he walked up to a six-month-old baby in its crib and put a gun to its head? Would that baby feel the same fear?" "Well of course not! But that baby does not know this is a life-threatening event" I replied.

"EXACTLY! That baby puts a different interpretation on that event then you do. The baby is lying there in its crib thinking, 'Oh goodie. That nice man is offering me a new toy. And that makes me happy!' So we have the same event — a gun to the head — but two different emotions. The baby feels joy and you feel fear."

He went on to say, "Imagine this despondent little man bent on committing suicide. He is marching resolutely toward the bridge from which he is going to leap to his death. All the way there he is saying to himself, 'I know this is wrong, and if I do it I may die and go to hell. But hell cannot be anything worse than what I am experiencing here and now. So please forgive me, God ... but I am going to do it!' Then just about that time, this robber slips up on him, puts this same gun to his head and says, 'Give me everything you have in your wallet and don't make a fast move or I will separate your head from your shoulders with this gun.' Do you think this suicidal man is going to cooperate with him? No! He is saying to himself, 'Oh, thank you God. You sent somebody to do this for me so that I do not have to do it for myself.' He makes a sudden move that guarantees the gun is going to go off and a bullet will pierce his skull."

There it is, friends ... THE SAME EVENT THREE TIMES. A gun to the head but a different reaction each time. I cringe in fear. The baby wiggles with joy. The suicidal man smiles in glorious relief. Three different emotions with the same event.

What makes the difference then? IT IS OUR INTER-PRETATION OF THE EVENT AND NOT THE EVENT ITSELF THAT DETERMINES WHAT EMO-TIONS WE EXPERIENCE. So then we have the power to determine what emotions we feel by the interpreta-tions we put on life's events. If we do not like what we feel we can give the event a different interpretation and experience a different emotion.

She says I am a stupid idiot and she can't stand to live with me anymore! I can give her the status of God Him-self Who knows me better than I know myself, and I can say she is right and I am an idiot. Or I can say, "That poor deluded soul! She does not know me at all. I am not stupid. I am not an idiot. And I will not give her the power over my life to determine how I feel about my intellectual prowess."

He says you are a helpless little nincompoop who can never make it alone. You can't afford to live apart from him. You can believe that and feel like a helpless little pawn. Or you can look at yourself realistically and say "I know better than that! I don't want to have to live alone, but if it comes to that I am a survivor. I will do whatever it takes to make it on my own. He is not the only fish in the pond, and I deserve something better than that!"

You can feel power and confidence instead of helplessness and powerlessness. BUT IT ALL DEPENDS ON YOU ... NOT WHAT IS HAPPENING TO YOU BUT WHAT INTERPRETATION YOU CHOOSE TO PUT ON THAT EVENT..

It is OK to feel whatever you are feeling. It is neither necessary nor helpful to deny what you are feeling. But if you are tired of feeling the way you do, the emotion can be changed by giving a different interpretation to that event.

AND THAT, MY FRIENDS, IS PUTTING THE POWER BACK IN **Y-O-U-R HANDS** WHERE IT REALLY BELONGS.

Next I offered an idea about:

HOW TO DEAL WITH FEAR

Several years ago my younger sister and my older sister's husband were killed in a horrible car/truck accident. The two couples were vacationing in Traverse City, Michigan where my older sister and her husband had a condominium. They had gone out to dinner and were returning from the restaurant. My younger sister was sitting in the passenger seat immediately behind the driver (my older sister's husband). Their spouses were sitting in the right hand side of the car.

As they approached the crest of a hill a truck was coming from the opposite direction with a low-boy trailer being towed behind his truck. Tragically, the trailer did not have air-brakes attached to the truck; the hitch was too big for the ball to which it was attached, and the weight of the earth-moving equipment it usually carried was not there to hold in on. The trailer was still coming up. It came off the hitch and careened immediately toward the car in which my sisters and brother-in-laws were riding.

The low-boy trailer first impacted their Chrysler at the front left headlight and simply stripped it to the floor all the way back to the right rear tail-light. There was no time to react. My brother-in-law in the right front seat said all he could remember was the sound like an explosion. When the dust and the shattered glass had settled, he was then where the back seat should have been. He was looking up into the sky because the roof of the car was no longer there. He looked over to the left side of the car where his wife had been, and there was nothing there. He knew instantly that she was gone. There was not enough left of the bodies of either my sister or brother-in-law to show in their closed caskets. My older sister was thrown into a forty-foot deep embankment, and one of her shoes was found thirty feet up in a tree.

After their funerals I remember riding around on our John Deere mower tractor watering the grass with my tears as I cut it. I was so angry at God! My sister was such a beautiful caring person with a ministry of her own. She was needed and all God had to do was let them out of that restaurant a few seconds before or a few seconds later. But no! God blew it ... and I was angry at Him for that. And I was telling Him so through my tears.

While riding on that tractor that day telling God how angry I was with Him, I heard Him ask of me: "What have you learned about ANGER?" I thought only a moment, then remembered what my mentor had taught me. "DR. FOSTER WILLIAMS TOLD ME THAT *ANGER FLOATS ON A SEA OF FEAR,* AND IF I WANT TO DISPEL THE ANGER IN MY LIFE I HAVE TO DEAL WITH THE FEAR." The voice of God came to me then: "He is right, you know. So son, what are you so afraid of?"

I remembered my brother-in-law standing before the closed casket of his wife. He was smiling, greeting people cheerfully, and recalling the good times he and my sister had had together. He was not evidently feeling sorry for himself. And I thought to myself, "If that was my wife lying there in that casket, I don't think I could stand it! I could never smile again like he was smiling."

Once again the voice of God came to me — "Is it possible, son, that you could be trusting that little lady a bit too much and Me not quite enough?" In that moment I came to the realization of that truth, dealt with the fear was plaguing me, and the anger quietly melted away.

We cannot rid ourselves of anger by denying its existence. We cannot rid ourselves of anger by promising ourselves we are not going to be angry anymore. WE CAN ONLY RID OURSELVES OF THE ANGER WE FEEL WHEN WE DEAL WITH IT HONESTLY ... BY FACING THE FEAR THAT IT FLOATS ON. When we deal courageously with the fear, the anger will disappear.

I concluded that session by emphasizing

THE FUTILITY OF SELF-PITY

It was evident from the start of the Divorce Recovery Workshop that he was not here to work the program. He was here to work the people. All he wanted in life was for people to feel sorry for him, and he played that one to the hilt.

A man in his mid-sixties, he had suffered the indignity of his first and only wife leaving him at that advanced age for another younger man. It was too great a blow to his self-esteem. He could not stand it. So for six weeks he moped, groveled for sympathy, and did little or nothing to work the program so that the program would work for him.

Six months later he was dead from a fast-growing cancer. Some of his friends from the class said to me, "Oh, isn't it awful that Mr. So-and-So died of cancer?" I knew these people well enough that I could say to them, "But he did not really die of cancer! He died a slow death of suicide. He didn't want to live anymore. He did not think he had anything worth living for. He set himself up to die. He turned on all the negative juices in his body that would work against him. Cancer got him ... but it really was a slow death of suicide."

When you inundate your body with "negative juices," you are asking for serious trouble. You could even kill yourself by doing that. You may be able to fool a few of your friends in the process, but you had better not fool yourself.

THE LUXURY OF SELF-PITY IS JUST TOO COSTLY FOR YOU TO OWN! IT COSTS SO MUCH AND IT GIVES YOU SO LITTLE IN RETURN. If you need to treat yourself to just a taste of that bitter stuff, you had better be careful. Get over your death wish.

5

SESSION THREE — "FORGIVENESS ... FINDING A NEW START IN LIFE"

We have discovered that this session is really the key in finally beginning to **GROW** through divorce. Only when people are able to come to the place of forgiveness are they able to mark the progress they have come to desire.

We began the session with the usual coffee and Get-Together, followed by the Show-And-Tell Time where people shared their excitement, progress, and sometimes their fears and concerns. Then came my Keynote address:

"FORGIVENESS ... AND FINDING A NEW START IN LIFE"

I am an avid tailgater... And for good reason! I love to read bumper stickers because some of the world's great wisdom can be found there. But I haven't mastered the art of reading the bumper stickers from ½ mile behind, so I tailgate. You know a person is a rank idiot if he puts his bumper stickers on the front bumper of his car because not many of us can read backwards through our rear-view mirrors to catch the message there.

Nevertheless I have discovered some great wisdom tailgating.

Recently I saw this one ... "God's retirement plan is out of this world."

Another one ... "Directions to heaven ... turn right and go straight."

But the best one I think I've ever seen is this ... "Christians aren't perfect ... they are just forgiven!"

The area of finding and experiencing forgiveness is one that so many people are reluctant to deal with ... and this includes people who are going through the trauma of divorce. This is tough. You can learn to toast your toast on mechanical level . You can learn to put in your storm windows, pay your bills, even do some rudimentary plumbing around the house. But to learn to forgive and to experience forgiveness is dealt with on a much deeper level and it is not that easy. Nevertheless, if you are going to grow through divorce rather than merely go through divorce, then this is one area you are going to have to deal with.

I think if I have said this once before but perhaps it needs to be said again. The church, the religious community, sometimes is awfully slow to exhibit a feeling of acceptance for those who have experienced divorce. Now or course the Bible doesn't teach that.in the minds of many that were stands out is the one on forgettable soon! At the conclusion of the last session of our Divorce Recovery Workshop, I am going to give each of you a copy over sermon I preached years ago about what everyone needs to know about divorce in which I trace the entire body of wisdom in the scripture that pertains to the divorce. I come to the conclusion that you have a right to remarry even with the blessing of scripture (and that may come as a surprise to many of you).

I believe there is a vast reservoir of puritanical prejudice in religion today that leads people to think that divorced people are permanently marred, bruised, tainted, condemned ... used articles no longer as good as new ones. If anything just ever happened to this lady sitting next to me with whom I have been married all these years, I would not look for some amateur who had never been married before. I would look for someone who had some experience that made them a better and wiser person.

But I just want to emphasize this. Whether or not the religious community or your church forgives you for whatever mistakes you have made, God has made provision for your forgiveness ... that is important ... and you must strive to forgive yourself as well.

A couple of sessions ago we talked about "time" healing the hurts of divorce. But only experiencing forgiveness gets the hate and the hurt out of your life permanently. Time may diminish it, but it doesn't totally heal it without forgiveness. And the good news of the Gospel is that GOD LOVES TO FORGIVE.

My favorite Bible verse follows immediately after John 3:16 ... it couples with it. John 3:16 reads: "For God so loved the world that he gave his only begotten son, that whosoever believeth in him should not perish, but have everlasting life." Then follows John 3:17 ... "For God sent not his son into the world to condemn the world, but that the world through him might be saved."

God did not send His Son Jesus Christ into the world to make us miserable ... to condemn us in our guilt ... but rather to forgive us and free us and save us from that unbearable burden of guilt.

One of my favorite stories in the New Testament is the story of the woman taken in the very act of adultery. Now, you see, the Old Testament Law was mighty touch on adulterers! Stone them ... stone them both to death.

That was the Old Testament prescription and remedy for this social ill. Kill them!

So the Scribes and Pharisees (enemies of Jesus) sought to trap him. They brought this little woman to Jesus and reminded him of what the Law of Moses said should be done to her. And then they asked him what He thought should be done to her. It was a trap and He knew it. If He said, "Kill her like Moses said," then the crowd would have forsaken Him as a merciless, unsympathetic legalist. But if He said, "Let her go," then the Scribes and Pharisees could say "Blasphemer! You have answered contrary to the Law of God.

I find it a little strange that these rulers of the Jews brought only this little woman who had been taken in the very act of adultery. That is a game that usually takes two to tango! But where was the man if they were taken in the very act? Their plot was evident to Jesus. They were out to get Him no matter what He answered.

So Jesus knelt down and wrote something in the sand. Who knows what He wrote? Maybe their names – maybe their sins – maybe the name of the one among them who was guilty of the same sin with this little woman. Then He looked up at them and said, "Let him who is without sin, CAST THE FIRST STONE AT HER." He knew who their stones were really aimed at ... at Him and not merely this little woman.

One by one there was sound of stones falling out of their fists onto the ground, and one by one they slipped away like whipped dogs with their tails behind their legs. And when they were all gone, Jesus looked up at this little woman with a tear-stained face and said, "Where are your accusers, Mam? Does no one condemn you?" She responded "No man, Lord." NOW HEAR THESE WORDS – "Neither do I condemn you" Jesus said. "Go and sin no more."

She was forgiven ... not condemned because of her human weakness ... because God is in the forgiving business. That is why His Son Jesus came to dwell among us.

Now let us face the facts. You made a promise ... you made a marriage vow ... "until death do us part" ... and you weren't able to keep that vow. Divorce is failure to meet God's standards for human relationships. God does not anybody to get hurt the way you have been hurt. That is why He established such tough standards for us to live by. But if we cannot or do not live up to those standards for whatever reasons, if we make mistakes that are fatal to our relationships, God does not quit loving us. He is ready and anxious to forgive us and offer us another chance in life. And how do we achieve that forgiveness? We simply confess our weakness and wrong-doing to Him, ask Him for help from now on, and accept His word that we are forgiven. When you do that, you are half-way home!

There is more? Yes, there is more! A second aspect of forgiveness may be even more difficult than saying "I'm sorry" to God. It is learning to forgive yourself. We have been programmed with this dumb idea that if we are not perfect, no one will love us. Isn't that crazy? HOW WOULD YOU FEEL IF YOU HAD TO LIVE IN THE PREESENCE OF SOMEONE WHO THOUGHT HE WAS PERFECT ALL THE TIME? I don't knowabout you, but I would feel inferior, unworthy, unlovely ... but God does not purpose that we feel that way. He sent not His Son into the world to condemn the world.

Many people live under the yoke of self-imposed guilt. They are unable to accept the fact that to be human means you will make mistakes. Until you experience the refreshing climate of self-forgiveness coupled with God's forgiveness ... until you can allow yourself the right top fail, you can never truly enjoy the humanity God has given as His good gift to you.

I want to add this caution. Forgiveness is not always an instant thing you grasp, but it is oftentimes something you grow into. And that is especially true when it comes to forgiving your ex-spouse for the things he or she has done to you. But remembering that none of us is perfect ... and that it is possible that we contributed at least a little bit to the demise of our relationship (and sometimes perhaps in ways we did not comprehend nor were we aware of), I have one other gigantic challenge which I want to offer you.

I HIGHLY RECOMMEND THAT WHEN YOU ARE FINALLY ABLE YOU GO TO YOUR EX-SPOUSE (if you have not already done something like this) AND SAY "I JUST WANT YOU TO KNOW HOW SORRY I AM. I REALIZE NOW I MADE MIS-TAKES AND I AM ASKING YOU TO FORGIVE ME FOR WHATEVER PART I PLAYED IN CONTRIBU-TING TO OUR DIVORCE. AND I OFFER YOU MY FORGIVENESS AS WELL!"

Hard? Incredibly hard! There is only one thing harder I could imagine for you and that is carrying that load of guilt around with you for the rest of your life. A GRUDGE IS A BURDEN TOO HEAVY FOR ANY TO BEAR. Let it go. Be done with it. Make the cut surgically clean. Let your ex-spouse know that the war is over, you aren't going to fight anymore, and that you just want both to go your separate ways and make the best of what life is ahead of you.

Just a couple of questions now and I will wrap this up. WHAT HAPPENS IF HE LAUGHS AT YOUR OFFER, SCORNS, RIDICULES, WANTS TO CARRY ON THE FIGHT? You don't have to do anything more. You have done your part! You have fulfilled your responsibility. And you are still clinging to a sickness if you feel the need to control other people's actions. You don't need to change them. You just need to change yourself in ways that you know are good for you. BUT I CAN'T FORGET WHAT HE DID TO ME. HOW CAN I EVER FORGET? The answer is you had better NOT forget. Those who forget go through the same thing all over again. Those who fail to learn the lessons history would teach us are condemned to live that history all over again. Don't forget. BEWARE! But don't be bitter and unforgiving and carrying a wound that never has a chance to heal.

One word of caution (and this is my last word to you). Animal psychologists (yes, there are actually such critters who study the behavior of animals with the hopes that this will give them some clues to human behavior) – Animal psychologists have observed a phenomenon which they call THE PUPPY DOG SYNDROME. You have probably witnessed this at one time or another. There is this little yappy dog that keeps snapping at the heels of this much bigger dog irritating the living daylights out of him. He tries to walk off and the little dog just keeps coming at him. The hair bristles on his neck, his ears stand straight up, he utters a guttural growl, and the puppy dog keeps coming.

Finally, when the big dog has had enough of this game, he turns around and starts at the little one like he is going to tear it apart. At that point the little dog rolls over on its back, puts its feet up in the air, bares his belly and lies there helplessly. The big dog snarls and growls over that bare belly like he is about to eat it up, asserts his dominance, and then finally walks away ... and the game is over.

If you have been playing "Puppy Dog" with your partner, yapping and nipping until he finally turns of you and threatens ... whereupon you roll over and play helpless ... he may be conditioned to see this as one more example of your playing the "Puppy Dog" game. You have got to assure him that this is not a game you are playing anymore. This is for real and you are dealing with things now on a rational (and not an emotional) basis.

When you have said it ... and meant it ... then you are ready for a new start in life.

GROUP DISCUSSION LED BY LA DONNA CHAMBERLIN

1. If you have experienced God's forgiveness in your divorce, describe how this came about and what brought you to this experience.

2. Where are you now in the struggle to forgive yourself?

3. If you have asked your ex-spouse for forgiveness, what happened? (If you have not, how do you feel about doing it?)

4. How are you handling the "forgetting" in your divorce?

5. What kind of relationship do you have today with the family into which you were born? How have they reacted to your divorce?

6. How did your divorce effect your ideas and feelings about family?

7. Do you presently feel accepted as a member of God's family? If so, how did yuou come to this feeling of acceptance?

MY PERSONAL GOAL FOR THIS WEEK IS:

We passed out two sheets dealing with forgiveness and divorce. See them in ADDENDUM 1 at the close of this book. They were:

1. Prayer For The Divorced

2. Dear Abby

ADDITIONAL NOTE

During the Class Discussion, one of the participants said "I could never forgive Ray for what he has done to me. He said if he ever saw me on the street he would spit in my face."

I said to her, "Betty Sue ... do you ever go to church?"
"Every Sunday" she replied.
"Do you ever say The Lord's Prayer in worship?"
"Every Sunday" she asserted.

"What do you do with that part of the prayer that says 'FORGIVE US OUR TRESPASSES *AS WE FORGIVE THOSE WHO TRESPASS AGAINST US*'?

Her unforgetable response: "Never thought about that before. Guess I will just skip that part from now on!"

At the next weekly session Betty Sue returned to tell us, "Well, I decided I would tell Ray I forgive him. But I could not tell him face to face and I was not going to talk to him on the telephone. So I wrote a note telling him I forgave him and gave it to my grandson to read before I sent it. The boy looked at its contents and then said to me, "Grandma, that is so fakey."

Neverless she finally came to the place where she could say she forgave him, and though Ray was an abusive alcoholic she remarried him (bad idea) and then divorced him again. But bless her heart, even though they were divorced she took care of him until the day he died. Somewhere along the line forgiveness must have occured.

6

SESSION FOUR — "HOW TO ASSUME RESPONSIBILITY ... FOR YOURSELF, YOUR CHILDREN, AND YOUR FUTURE"

By this time we are beginning to see real progress in the lives of many of our participants. Enthusiasm and participation is growing. Many seem eager to get on with the program and some report that they are meeting with other participants during the week to share with them.

After the Coffee and Informal Get-Together and the Show-And-Tell Time I offered the Key-Note Address entitled:

"HOW TO ACCEPT RESPONSIBILITY ... FOR YOURSELF, YOUR CHILDREN, AND YOUR FUTURE."

One of the desperate (and futile) searches for a lot of single adults is the search to find somebody out there who will make them happy again. If you are into blaming somebody else for your unhappiness, then you will probably be into making someone else responsible for your happiness as well. That is a tender trap ... and it is a fatal trap as well.

No one in all the world is responsible for your happiness except yourself. The truth is NO ONE CAN MAKE YOU HAPPY ANYMORE THAN ANYONE CAN MAKE YOU ANGRY OR HURT OR SAD ... OR ANYTHING ELSE. We learned in the second session that the things that happen to us are not the direct cause of our feelings, but rather our interpretation of those events as we see them. (R.E.T. — Rational Emotive Therapy) — remember it? You and I choose our own emotions by the interpretations we put on whatever is happening around us. We can change those emotions by changing our interpretations of those events.

The temptation is to think that if we can just find the right person the next time around, then we can be happy again. I need to tell you that is very dangerous thinking. IF YOU CAN'T BE HAPPY WHERE YOU ARE, THEN YOU CAN'T BE HAPPY WHERE YOU AIN'T!

If you do not find happiness before you enter into a new relationship, then that relationship is probably going to be doomed to the same sort of destructive stuff you suffered through in your latest heartbreak.

It is easy to go on blaming someone else for your misery or lack of happiness, but that only prolongs the agony. Each of us only gets one shot at life ... one time around is the quota for us all.

(Have you heard about the two fellows who were discussing reincarnation? One said to the other, "I believe we keep; coming back to earth until we are finally perfect!" The other responded with a groan, "Oh no ... This is probably my last time around!")

Since it is quite evident that one time around is all we get, it is important not to waste life on garbage that does us no good at all. We must learn to take responsibility for ourselves ... for our children (if we have any of them) ... and for our future as well.

You can begin by assuming responsibility for your part in the failure of your marriage. That is what last week's theme was all about. You don't even have to be the major contributing factor in the demise of that relationship. But because we are less than perfect human beings, it is all right to say "O.K. I goofed. I could have done better. I should have done better. And I am truly sorry for that. Please forgive me ... and know that I forgive you as well."

The problem with playing the BLAME GAME is that nobody ever gets to win that one. You cannot relive the years of your marriage and changed what is now history. But you can accept responsibility for your part in the failure of your history and thereby change your future.

People do not divorce SITUATIONS. They divorce PEOPLE WHO CREATE SITUATIONS and then fail to take responsibility for those situations.

Assuming responsibility for yourself means starting with your past and putting that into perspective. It means expressing your responsibility for the failures in your marriage to your ex-spouse. NOW HERE IS THE GOOD NEWS. If both parties will do this, then the blame game will cease and post-marital relationships will not have to be a continual war. Some of you are really longing for something like that, aren't you? (Well no — some of you would like to see the old buzzard fry in his or her own grease for awhile. You have got to see them suffer awhile before you are going to be willing to change.)

Well that is all right (I guess) if you are content to continue to be miserable. But sooner or later you may just tire of it. When you do, then maybe — just maybe — you may choose to get on with living. I hope you do. But you don't do that by rehashing the past. You let go of the past and start living in the present.

Having chosen to accept responsibility for your past, then you must also accept responsibility for your present situation as well. Quite often we hear people blame their present situation on their past. "If it wasn't for that old so-and-so, I wouldn't be living in this dump. But you see that is not quite the whole truth. You chose to be totally dependent on him for much too much of your own life. Perhaps you did not take the opportunity to get a good education to prepare yourself for a meaningful life. You sacrificed that in order to be cared for by him. Perhaps you chose to have all those expensive kids. But you made a choice that enabled all of that to happen. Perhaps nobody told you this before, but I will tell you this now. Every little child born today is going to cost his parents an average of $250,000 (a quarter of a million dollars) by the time he leaves home and finishes college.

Sometimes we make decisions without counting the cost. When the results of those decisions come crashing down on you, burying your nose in the boob-tube is not going to get the job done for you. Bar-hopping or pill-popping is not going to make things any better for you. You can go on blaming someone else and pitying yourself as long as you wish. But is it really a satisfying goal in life to accumulate a whole warehouse full of "I'm so sorry's" or would you rather get on with building a worthwhile life?

Being responsible means that you face up to your responsibilities serously. It means that you plan to assume these responsibilities in an organized and intelligent way, and that you execute that plan. The world is already overpopulated with people who are willing to fix the blame on someone or something else. To be responsible means that we are no longer interested in fixing the blame but rather fixing the problem. As Nike puts it, "JUST DO IT!"

A second area of responsibility for many of you will be that of CARING FOR YOUR CHILDREN. Divorce is as frightening and devastating to those little tykes as it is to you. Some of them may respond to the bad news with sobs of terror. By the way ... your children probably knew about that deteriorating relationship long before you did. You probably ignored the strange looks your partner shot in your direction ... but they didn't. You probably passed off lightly the arrogant tone in your partner's voice, but they caught it and felt it and knew that "something was rotten in Denmark" long before you were willing to acknowledge it. You see, we don't want to believe this is happening to us so we just shove it aside sometimes until it cannot be ignored anymore.

That leads me to this observation: I have seen so many marriage relationships that simply "endured" until the children were gone from the nest, and then the relationship terminated. "We stayed together for the kids," they explain. Well that is not a good enough reason for staying together in a bad marriage because the kids know what is going on. They can sense it. They can feel it. They can smell it. And we are not doing them a great favor in pretending things are just fine when they are rotten as all get-out.

Part of being adult is accepting responsibility for the children that are a part of our lives. Divorce never makes things any easier of the budget (except on the lawyer's budget). There is quite often the aggravation of limited finances, even more limited time for the children than was available before because now your time is at a premium. There is the added pressure on the custodial parent who is stuck with the kids most of the time. It is not easy. It is in all reality a tough life. But there are some guidelines Jim Smoke offers in his book and LaDonna is going to lead you in them in just a few minutes.

But finally, if you are going to grow through divorce rather than merely go through divorce, you have to **ASSUME RESPONSIBILITY FOR YOUR FUTURE.** Some of you may be wondering "My Future? I have no future! What kind of a future is there out there for me?" You are not weird if that thought has crossed your mind a time or two. We have discovered in our previous workshops that 90% of the people have contemplated suicide at one time or another. 50% of them have been able to talk about it right off the top. Another 40%

are not quite so vocal but we can read between the lines and catch that they too have been thinking about it. It isn't much of a solution to their problems, but at least they think about it.

A gun ... drugs ... a car wrapped around a tree ... there are numerous ways to get that horrible deed done. But as we shared with you previously, to inundate your body with the negative juices that accompany constant nagging negative emotions is to do yourself in the slow way. Destroy the immune system in your body and you are going to die. The white cell count in our blood, the part that fights disease, is crippled and reduced when we are depressed or constantly angry or fearful or hopeless.

But we know that when a person has a sense of purpose in life, a reason for being and living, a positive self-image that confirms the worthiness of his or her existence, the white blood cell count goes up. So you do have a future. The future is as bright as the promises of God.

But you can kill it, destroy it, maim and cripple it by refusing to plan for the future and take control over it. IF YOU HAVE SOMETHING WORTHWHILE TO DO, SOMETHING TO LOOK FORWARD TO AND SOMEONE TO LOVE WHO LOVES YOU, YOUR FUTURE IS LIMITLESS.

When it comes to planning for the future, there are basically three kinds of people. There are those who are content to WATCH THINGS HAPPEN. There are those who DON'T EVEN PAY ATTENTION to know what is happening. And there are those who MAKE THINGS HAPPEN. The future is satisfying only to those persons who decide they will take the responsibility for their own future and make things happen.

Bob Schuller is fond of saying, 'IF YOU FAIL TO PLAN, THEN YOU PLAN TO FAIL.' Future planning begins by honestly assessing the present. Be honest with yourself. The last person you ought to try to fool is yourself. As the poet put it, *"To thine own self be true ... and it shall follow as the night the day, thou canst then be false to no man."* Don't try to fool yourself. Honestly assess where you are right now. Your life style may have to change. You may have to get a different job. You may have to go to school and upgrade your abilities. You may have to take inventory of your talents and move in another more satisfying direction. But you can do any of these things if only you are determined and you try.

Having a job means putting in time and getting pay for your effort. Having a career means having identity, respect, prestige and remuneration. Having a job means merely DOING something. Having a career means BEING something. Divorce in your life may be the very impetus that makes it possible for you to have a whole new start in an entirely new direction in life (if that is something that appeals to you). Look at this divorce as an opportunity for personal; growth rather than merely a roadblock on your plans toward going nowhere.

For a moment let's try to imagine the worst. Suppose Iran or North Korea or Al Qaeda becomes able to bring their threats to this country and they drop a nuclear bomb on Indianapolis. Everything around us is devastated. Utilities are no longer available. We can't get gasoline in our cars even if there were roads good enough to drive on. Schools, factories, stores, hospitals are closed. Could you survive?

If you had someone who needed you or some worthwhile purpose in life, you not only could survive. You would be hell-bent to do so! You are survivors. So you can survive the tragedy that has hit you and your family. Establishing goals and then reaching them reinforces this message: "I AM SOMEBODY WORTHWHILE, AND I AM GOING SOMEWHERE!" Many look on an unhappy marriage where commitments were not kept and decide they will never make commitments again. They become "commitment shy" because they have been burned ... they have been hurt.

It is the easiest thing in the world to build a shrine around the hurt in your life and worship at that shrine for the rest of your miserable life. But this much is certain if you do that ... You will not enrich your life at that altar. You will not lengthen your life ... you will shorten it there. you will not find much joy in a sick sort of religion like that.

I pray that each of you will make the decision to take responsibility for yourself, your children, and your future. But no one can make those decisions for you. Even if I was able, I would not do that for you because I respect every one of you too much. IT IS YOUR LIFE TO DO WITH IT WHATEVER YOU WANT . I can only hope that you will have the sense to take responsibility for it and do something with your life while you still have the opportunity. I have prayed to that end. I have tried to put feet to those prayers by sharing with you evening after evening. And now the rest is up to you.

GROUP DISCUSSION LED BY LA DONNA CHAMBERLIN

1. What are some of the areas of failure in your marriage for which you are willing to accept responsibility? (Please do not force it ... share only if you are ready.)

2. What are some of the struggles you are having in assuming responsibility for your present situation?

3. Are your goals set by you, or are they "contingency goals" that are dependent upon other people and other events or situations?

4. What is the biggest problem you face in being a parent?

5. What kind of picture of your ex-spouse do you present to your children?

6. If you knew you could not fail, what would you like to attempt to do? What would you like to attempt to be?

7. What is your attitude about your future?

At this point we passed out Jim Smoke's GUIDE-LINES FOR SUCCESSFUL PARENTING (See Addendum Three).

Then I shared a discovery I had made called

SCRIPTING

Let's back up a couple of weeks and review where we have come from. Our first night we talked about emotions. We established first that whatever emotions you experienced (no matter how negative they seemed to be) it was all right to have them. The important factor is not what emotions you experience, but what you do with them. We also emphasized that it is not what happens to you that determines your emotions, but rather what interpretation you put on the events that triggered those emotions. So you can change your emotions if you wish by changing your interpretation that you put on the events that preceded those emotions.

The second night we talked about how we can deal with the emotions we have about our ex-spouses. We tried to isolate those emotions that were strongest in our lives, and they led us to a better understanding of what went wrong in our marriage (the seven basic causes of divorce) and how we must avoid those mistakes in our future relationships.

There is another thing I believe is vital to understand as we think about our relationship with others. It is the thing that psychologists call "**SCRIPTING**". I first learned about Scripting when I was Senior Minister at Corydon Old Capitol United Methodist Church where I served for 14 years. The Rev. Vernon Nossett was our Counseling Minister on our staff there.

Vernon grew up in a preacher's house. His dad was a "Jack-Leg" preacher ... just up from the coal mines and began preaching without a whole lot of education or preparation. His was a very negative style not only in his preaching but in his raising a family.

He told his son Vernon that he was to be seen and not heard, that he would never amount to anything much at all (which was probably a reflection of his own negative self-image). So Vernon went on the college and did very well. Then on to seminary where he graduated Magna Cum Laude (I never had that problem!). But that was problematic to him because he could not equate this success with what his father had been telling him all his life.

Vernon eventually was appointed Program Director of the Henryville Boys School (a home for delinquent boys) in Southern Indiana. He established a program so significant there that representatives from like institutions throughout the United States were coming to him to find out why his program was so successful. The rate of recidivism among his charges was astoundingly better than anywhere else around. And that was a problem to Vernon because his dad had taught him that he would never amount to much and would never succeed at anything he tried to do.

We had a place down on Rough River Lake in Kentucky and we invited Vernon and his wife down there to stay with us for awhile. One beautiful Summer evening we were sitting out in the front yard talking about our work and he introduced the concept of Scripting to me. He informed me that SOMEWHERE BETWEEN THE AGE OF TWO AND FOUR, MOST OF US ARE SCRIPTED. We get an idea of who and what we are and what we are supposed to be doing for the rest of our lives, and then it is like WE GO ON STAGE AND PLAY THAT ROLE FOR THE REST OF OUR LIVES (or at least until we consciously do something about it).

He described his Scripting Role as a **"NO-BE SCRIPT"**. He could not please his father no matter what he did. And whenever he succeeded it distressed him and confused him because he could not reconcile it with his Script.

I asked him how I could discover my Script. He told me that we need to dig as far back in our consciousness as we can. Bring up the earliest memories of our childhood. Try to remember what our favorite stories were. Try to remember who our most memorable teacher was.

Try to remember what we learned from some impressive authority figure in our lives.

He set me on a journey of intense inward inspection that literally consumed me for a period of 24 hours. I could think about little else than trying to recall the earliest memories that were hidden deep in my consciousness. I remembered that my favorite stories were the Frank Merriwell stories … particularly where the baseball player came to the 9th inning with his team down three runs. Bases were loaded when he came to bat and there were two outs. The pitcher ran the count to three balls and two strikes. And the next throw came right down the middle of the plate and he hit it out of the park for a grand-slam home run and the ball game was won. I played that game in my own mind innumerable times while I was growing up.

After a lot of searching, a strange memory floated back into my mind with the force of a gigantic jolt of electricity. I had not even thought about this for perhaps thirty years. I was a little boy again … crying because of some mishap that occured in my life … and my mother would draw my head up to her tummy, hold me close, and say these exact words — "There, there, now son … EVERYTHING IS GOING TO BE ALL RIGHT!" "EVERYTHING … E-V-E-R-Y-T-H-I-N-G …EVERYTHING IS GOING TO BE ALL RIGHT!"

And the message I took from that was ALWAYS ...
EVERYTHING ... WOULD TURN OUT ALL
RIGHT IN THE END (like my baseball games for
instance). What I got from this script was that I could be
the world's greatest procrastinator and it would still
work out all right in the end. If it wasn't going well now,
heck — it is only the seventh inning. We have got two
more innings after this and we can pull it out in the end
just like Frank Merriwell did!

That was A POSITIVE SCRIPT but it could cause a
lot of trouble. We built a church 9 yards short of a football field long down there in Corydon ... a magnificent,
beautiful structure. It is longer than a football field now.
They have prospered and added to it. But while we were
planning for this new structure, I kept assuring myself
and others around me that our good people always
responded affirmatively whenever they saw a genuine
need. So we kept adding on and on and on until we got
past 1/2 million dollars indebtedness. Back there in
1974, that was a lot of money for people in a town of less
that 3000 people. Then some of our leadership said "We
think that is enough for now."

My overly optimistic Script enabled me to be a procrastinator and sometimes unrealistic about what could
and should be done. I've changed my Script only slightly.
I have rid myself of the "EVERYTHING" in that Script. I
am still a flaming optimist. In fact, I was the charter Pres-

ident of the Optimist Club there in Corydon. And I still subscribe to the creed of that service club. But I have learned my limitations over time and I am now able to recognize that Scripting Voice when it rears its voice in my mind. I can now order my life in a more reasonable and satisfactory manner.

EACH OF YOU WERE SCRIPTED. I don't know what your Script may be. But if you can recognize some of the patterns of behavior in your lives, and some of those voices that compel you to think and act the way you do subconsciously, then you may well on the way to recognizing what went wrong in your relationship. And what is even more important, you are well on the way to seeing that it will never happen to you again.

7

SESSION FIVE — "HEY, GOD ... WHAT DO I DO WITH SEX?"

The usual Coffee and Informal Get-Together began the fifth session, again followed by the Show-and-Tell Time where participants shared their progress in Goal-Setting. Then followed the Keynote Address entitled:

"Hey, God ... What Do I Do With Sex?"

At the close of each previous Divorce Recovery Workshop, we asked the participants to help us by evaluating what we have done with them. We ask three basic questions:

1. What was the most helpful to you in this DRW"
2. What was least helpful to you in this DRW?

3. What would you do differently if you were conducting your own DRW?

The responses have been most affirmative (BLESS THEIR LITTLE HEARTS)! If they had not been so gracious, we probably would have given up long ago. We are grateful for the encouragement we have received ... but we are also grateful for the suggestions and guidance they have offered to enrich this program even more.

One of the suggestions given to us had to do with dealing with the problem of being a single adult trying to handle those sometimes anxious sexual drives. This evidently is a real problem to many who have known the joys of sex in the context of a marital relationship, and then have had that legitimate avenue of appropriate sexual expression denied them. So in response to this suggestion by some of your fellow sufferers from way back, we are going to try to deal with this important question:

"Hey, God ... What Do I Do With Sex?"

The place I want to begin is with an affirmation of what my Christian faith has to say to me about my own human sexuality. I must confess that I have come a long way in the journey of understanding of myself and how God created me and why He made me the way He did.

I grew up in a home where "sex" was a nasty word. We did not talk about it. Nice little Christian boys didn't even think about it (and that meant that frequently I was not a nice Christian boy because I thought a lot about sex). It was evident however that somebody around that house was thinking about sex because there were seven of us kids growing up in that family. My brother and I each had five sisters. (That still only spells seven ... Are you still with me?) :-) I am not complaining about my parents and our sex education. They did the best they could with the little learning they had, but I think it was just not sufficient.

The Victorian Puritanical atmosphere in which I was raised did not jibe real well with life, however. So I began to investigate the Scriptures more deeply. It is actually surprising what the Bible has to say when you read it for yourself instead of taking uncritically and a face value what other people are telling you it says (and informing you what you MUST believe). I want to encourage you to read your Bible. Sometimes it can be a fascinating book ... and sometimes it can be a terribly dull and dry book too! But I commend it to you for your own reading and personal growth.

One of the first things I learned about the Bible is that it is a real 'SEXY' book. It is filled with references to sex (but I must add) in a wholesome way. I found out as I read the Creation Story in Genesis One that after God finished creating Adam and Eve (man and woman, male and female), He stood back, surveyed His handiwork, smiled and said, "AH, THAT'S VERY GOOD" (Genesis

1:31). There stood God's creative masterpiece ... man and woman ... standing NAKED in the Garden of Eden. And God looked at them in their nakedness and said to Himself, "AH, THAT'S VERY GOOD!"

God made you and me this way ON PURPOSE! He made us sexual beings. Sex is one of God's great gifts to you and me. I dare say we have no right whatsoever to disparage any of the gifts that He has given us. So I had to make a choice. Should I believe and accept the wisdom of those around me who were proclaiming that "Sex is bad"? Or should I accept the witness of the Holy Scriptures and the testimony of God Himself that "AH, THAT IS VERY GOOD"? Well I think you know pretty well where I came out on that one.

Think about this for a minute. If God created me with a stomach that craves food (incidentally He did that very thing) and then the first time I started to put food into my mouth He jumped on me and said, "AHHH... AHHH...AHHH — Sinner boy, nice people don't do nasty things like eat food," — I would have to wonder what sort of a wierd God is it Who created me this way. Wouldn't you do the same?

If God created me with lungs that hunger desperately for air, but then said to me the first time I tried to breathe, "NASTY! NASTY! NASTY! YOU SHOULDN'T EVEN THINK ABOUT BREATHING!" then I think I would have a hard time understanding, appreciating, loving or even trusting a Creator like that. How about you?

Now very deeply a part of my human nature is my human sexuality. That is God's good gift to me. My sexual drives, my sexual energies, my very sexual nature is God's give to me, and if God looks at that part of me which He created and says, "AHHH ... THAT IS GOOD" then I have no right to look at myself and say, "AHHH ... THAT IS VERY BAD."

The hunger for sex in God's creation is sometimes as strong as our hunger for food or air, and only a fiend would create me that way and then say "Don't eat, don't breathe, and don't yield to your sexual appetites."

AM I SAYING THEN THAT ANYTHING GOES? THAT YOU CAN HAVE SEX ANY TIME YOU WANT IT? THAT GOD DOESN'T CARE ABOUT THAT? **ABSOLUTELY NOT!** God demands that each of these human appetites are to be used for the purposes He created them. God does not take pleasure in seeing us distort the appetite for food so that we live to eat instead of eating to live. God is not delighted to see us hyperventilate. In fact, yhou over-indulge in ingesting air and you are going to pass out. God made you so that too much air too fast is going to get you in trouble.

Likewise God is not over-joyed when we take the good gift of human sexuality and use it in some ways He never intended. So the important question is, "For what purpose did He create us as sexual beings?" I believe our human sexuality is a gift from God for TWO BASIC PURPOSES.

One is for procreation. "Be fruitful and multiply" he told that first pair in the Garden of Eden. There are a lot of commandments the human race has chosen to ignore, but this is not one of them! We have over-populated this globe in many places, and it is about time we relaxed a little bit when it comes to obeying this commandment.

There is a second purpose designed into our human sexuality. God has created both men and women with an additional bonus in their sexual natures. Without any intention of procreation, we can enjoy the ecstasies of sex. A woman's ability to experience orgasm as well as man has absolutely nothing to do with procreation. It has only to do with the joy of man and woman experiencing a "oneness" that is incomparable to any other experience in life. That is God's gift to the human race that was not given to the animal kingdom. We alone, of all God's creation, are made to express mutual love in sex that is satisfying to both male and female.

I happen to believe that procreation is the least important of the two purposes in sex. Expressing genuine love for one another is the higher and greater purpose in human sexuality. But the joys of sex, God says, are to be reserved for marriage. The priceless gift of human sexuality is too sacred to be wasted on someone who does not express love and total commitment in that act. The emotional involvement that is related to the act of sex spells heartbreak for the person who is then denied the commitment that act implies, and it spells debilitation for the man or the woman who drags it through the mud as though it has little or no significance at all —WHO SAYS 'WHAM! BAM! THANK YOU, MAM!" and then slithers on to his next conquest without any understanding of how sacred the act of sex must be!

I have talked in my office with men, single adults, who have told me: "I have gone to bed with a different woman every night of the week, and it just is not there. I'm not happy. I'm not fulfilled. I'm not satisfied! What is wrong with me?" The answer to that question every time is SEX CAN NEVER BE THE SATISFYING EXPERIENCE GOD DESIGNED IT TO BE FOR YOU IF IT IS TREATED CASUALLY AND WITHOUT AN UNEQUIVOCAL COMMITMENT OF ONE PARTNER TO THE OTHER FOR ALL TIME.

We dare not sell this beautiful gift short! Use it the way God intended it and it can be for you the most fulfilling experience of your life. Abuse it and degrade it and it will be for you at best a temporary pleasure that soon loses its thrill and the joy it was intended to bring.

All right now ... let me enter your minds for just a moment. Some of you may be thinking "This may all be true. But I still have this deep and irrepressible drive within me that longs for me to be in somebody else's arms, to share all of me with them. And this drive doesn't go away. So what am I going to do with it? What kind of help can you offer me?

To begin, it will help you to look at love and sex in what I am going to call "the Christian context" rather than in "the Animal context." WE ARE NOT MERE ANIMALS. We are special creations by God. Do you want sex to be nothing more than the expression of the animal instincts within you? Do you want to be the sort of licentuous person who says with the rest of the animal kingdom, "I WANT WHAT I WANT WHEN I WANT IT" and "ANYBODY WHO STANDS IN MY WAY IS GOING TO GET HURT." That acceptance of instant gratification is the very mark of gross immaturity.

You have a decision to make about how you are going to relate to God's plan for your life. God comes out pretty plain and certain against adultery and fornication. Why? Not because He wants you to be miserable, but because He wants to spare you the horrible hurt of BEING MISERABLE!

Secondly, I know that doesn't make the drive go away. It is still there. So what are we to do with it if we have no legitimate sexual partner with whom we can share it? Some people believe masturbation is the answer to that problem. Frankly I do not see any prohibition of this in the Scripture. Yet I doubt that this is a complete solution to the problem. For some it may be a temporary relief, but it does not make the problem go away for long. What underlies our sexual desires is this intense need to be loved and to love. You can't give that to yourself in masturbation. It doesn't solve the problem.

Some say cold showers are the perfect answer to the problem. I would hate to have to pay the water bill of some of you who hold this belief!

And what about SUBLIMATION? We all learned that word as teenagers, didn't we? We sublimate our energies by redirecting them .. using your sexual energies like coaching little league baseball or being a gray lady working in the hospital. I am not sure that this is the perfect solution to the problem either. How many people do you know who play baseball at midnight? How many hospitals let sex-crazed gray ladies roam their halls at midnight when their patients are supposed to be asleep?

St. Paul offered a partial answer to this problem that I am not convinced is the end-all solution to this problem either. He said, "To the unmarried and to widows I say this: It is a good thing if they stay as I am myself (single); but if they cannot control themselves, they should marry. Better be married than burn wth vain desire." (I Corinthians 7:8,9).

The problem with this approach is that we get ourselves in worse hot water by prematurely going out and choosing a new marriage partner without being certain that this isreally the one we want and need and can live with for the rest of our lives. Anytime you enter into a desperate marriage relationship without the ultimate in commitment, you are going to end up with a far worse problem than learning how to control your sexual desires. Don't jump into another relationship just because you need a bed-partner. You need a better reason for marriage than that.

But if you can look at these tremendous appetites for sex and love that God has given you, recognize the beauty of these gifts, and then remind yourself that you are going to use these gifts for their highest intended purpose when the right person comes into your life. YOU CAN HANDLE YOUR SEX DRIVES. You can handle them. You are not going to be dead sexually, but you can handle those desires and impulses when you have set your priorities on how they will be used.

I say YOU CAN HANDLE YOUR SEX DRIVES because you do that all the time practically every day. Fellows, you see a pretty girl walking down the street and you don't jump her right there on the sidewalk and do your thing. Gals, you see a particularly good-looking fellow in the office where you work, and you don't jump on his desk, do a strip-tease, and do your thing right there in public. You can and you do exhibit a sense of self-control every day. So don't deny your strength. It is there. You can't deny it. Just continue to use it as you know you should.

Now let me ask you a question that perhaps has never been posed to you before. WHAT DO YOU THINK WENT THROUGH THE MIND OF JESUS WHEN HE SAW A PRETTY GIRL WALKING DOWN THE STREET? The Scripture says that "He was tempted in all points like as we are, YET WITHOUT SIN." (Hebrews 4:15)

Jesus was fully human as well as fully divine. To me that means that He enjoyed the sight of a beautiful girl. He never sought to seduce her or rape her. No, I think He looked at the beautiful girls of His day, admired their beauty, and said "OOOOOOH-LA-LA, GOD! YOU CERTAINLY GOT THOSE MOLECULES TOGETHER IN AN ATTRACTIVE FASHION! SHE IS REALLY NICE TO LOOK AT." And then He went on His way.

When you go to an Art Gallery and see a beautiful painting, you don't sneak around until the guard and all the art patrons are out of sight, then find a way to sneak that painting off the wall, under your coat, out the door so you can take it home and hang it in your bedroom. No, you admire it — admit its beauty — thank God for it. And then you go on your way. YOU DON'T HAVE TO POSSESS IT IN ORDER TO ENJOY IT. (And if you do, then you have a sickness you need to deal with before you get yourself in another relationship. That is a part of the garbage in your life that has to go.

So here is a part of the problem we have with this sexual nature of ours. If we have a distorted view of our own self-worth, then we resort to making collections of things to show other people how important we are. It is sophomoric, high-schoolish, immature to think that people are going to love and respect us if we can lay so many trophies, so many conquests, so many sex partners on our list of accomplishments.

We do not have to possess another beautiful person in order to enjoy their beauty. We fellows here tonight appreciate the way you girls present yourselves so attractively. We can look and admire and then walk off without any need to possess you because we respect you as persons and not merely objects to be conquered for our own sick needs. If you are not at that point in your personal development yet, then a part of the garbage you need to be dealing with is your own self-image and why it is so important to be so possessive and to use people solely for your own ego-needs.

Now I have been on occasion accused of being naive, but I think I am awake enough to know that several (if not many) of you have been struggling with this Christian ideal of sex as I have been describing it. And if you are not struggling with it now, you probably will be struggling with it sometime in the future. And there may be some of you who have not been able to live up to this ideal. What can I say to you?

The first thing I want to say is that Jesus has some good things to say to you. The first thing He has to say is "I'm not nearly so hung up on the sin of sexual impropriety as most of you are." Look at the story of THE PRODIGAL SON in the New Testament. The stupid young fellow demanded his share of his inheritance evern before his father died. And the father gave it to him. He promptly went out into a far country and wasted his money on wine, women and song ... "riotous living" the Scripture describes it. (Not "righteous" but "riotous" living.)

Finally when he was broke and hungry, he came to his senses and realized the servants in his father's house had it better than he did. So he went back home with the intention of asking his father just make him one of his servants. But the father welcomed him with open arms and fully accepted him again. Now this would have been a wonderful opportunity for Jesus to indulge in a lecture about the evils of sexual wantonness. But He didn't — not a word about that. Just the wonderful message that the son had been lost but now was found.

On another occasion Jesus confronted a woman at Jacob's Well who had had five husbands and the man she was living with was not even her husband then. Here was an opportunity to present a great lecture on unfaithfulness, but He blew it! Not a word about her sexual transgressions.

I've already told you that beautiful story of the woman who was taken in the very act of adultery and brought to Jesus. Did he condemn her? Absolutely not! He said, "Neither do I condemn you, Go and sin no more."

So I am telling you that society places a whole lot more weight on sexual sins that Jesus did. Oh yes — He calls sin "sin" - but He is not all strung out about it. We tend to think that adultery or fornication is one of the most unforgivable sins people can commit. But that was a sin that Jesus had no problem handling and forgiving when one was honest and open in their confession about it.

If you have failed ... or if you are failing now or even fail in the future ... give yourself a break. Admit your weakness. Confess it to God Who truly cares about you as His child. Ask Him to help you live in such a way that this beautiful gift will not lose any of its luster or beauty by dragging it through the mud of human experience that approaches that of the animal kingdom.

Now I want to close with one of my favorite stories. It is a true story. Once there was a Bishop in the Roman Catholic Church who name was SIN ... BISHOP SIN. His colleagues used to joke with him. "What if you ever becomne elevated to the position of Cardinal in the Church? Then you would be "Cardinal Sin!" The truth of the matter is he eventually was elevated to that high office in the Church.

But while he was still Bishop, he learned about a little nun in his diocese who was reporting that she had these vivid visions of the living Christ. He was not sure whether those visions were authentic of whether perhaps she was losing touch with reality. So he called her into his office and questioned her about those visions. She described in intimate detail the visions she had of the living Christ. And the Bishop was not sure from this conversation whether these visions were authentic or not.

So he asked her, "Sister, do you think you will ever have any more visions of this living Christ?" 'Oh, without question, I know I shall" she responded. "Will you do me a small favor if you have another vision of the living Christ?" he asked her. "Anything you desire, Bishop. What can I do?" Bishop Sin said to this little nun, "Sister, the next time you see the living Christ, ask him this question: 'WHAT WAS THE BISHOP'S CHIEF SIN BEFORE HE BECAME A BISHOP?'" Aha ... what a smart question! He knew that only God and his Confessor would know the answer to that question.

A few months later it was reported that the little nun was at it again ... rep;orting those stories about more visions of the living Christ. So he called her back in and asked her about her latest visions. She described them in infinite detail. Then he said, "Oh by the way, Sister ...

just by the way ... did you remember to ask the living Christ the question I gave you?" "I did! I did!" she replied. "And what did He answer?" the Bishop inquired.

"I said to the living Christ, 'WHAT WAS THE BISHOP'S CHIEF SIN BEFORE HE BECAME A BISHOP?' And the Christ answered me: 'THE BISHOP'S CHIEF SIN BEFORE HE CAME A BISHOP WAS ... IT WAS ... I CAN'T REMEMBER IT ANYMORE."

That is the kind of God I come to proclaim to you today. In all of our weakness ... in all of our failings ... we can bring it to Him. He paid the price for our sins. And when we give it to Him, He removes our sin from us as far as the East is from the West. He remembers it no more.

So do not despair if you have been unable to live up to the highest ideal of love and sexuality as God intends it. Give it to God. Ask Him to help you. Then pick up the pieces and go in the strength He offers you to live a new and better life.

GROUP DISCUSSION QUESTIONS

1. Is there such a thing as "the Christian view" of sex?
2. If you have a different view, where does it come from? How does it help you? Would you recommend it to others?

3. Is society doing anything to help you handle the problems of being single, or are they doing anything to complicate your problem?

4. Keith Miller in *Sexual Choices For Singles* lists seven popular (or not so popular) ways of handling the sex drives. Are any of these helpful to you?

❈ Repression and denial of the sexual drive

❈ Suppression and sublimation

❈ Platonic friendships

❈ Fantasizing

❈ Masturbation

❈ Sex with an unmarried person

❈ Sex with a homosexual or lesbian person

5. Why do you think society is so "hung up" on sex? Or are we about as we should be?

6. Did your parents do a good job teaching you about sex and love?

7. What will your children say about your teaching them of sex/love?

(An interesting addition to this presentation) — We never allow two ex-spouses to attend the same sessions. It might inhibit them from being as open as is necessary, and the purpose of our Divorce Recovery Workshops is not to get divorcees back together but to enable them to discover help so that they may never have to go through divorce again.

However we had one couple that expressed a desire to attend the workshop together. At the time we were conducting one of the workshops in Carmel where they were both living, and the other workshop in Fishers. So I suggested that she would be welcome to attend the sessions in her home town and he could come to Fishers for our workshop there.

When we inquired in the discussions that followed the presentation of sex, she boldly proclaimed "I think this is some of the most outdated and wrong information you could offer. I played around with sexual partners before I got married and I will surely do it again." I asked if she had any children and when they came of age what would she tell them about how to conduct themselves in this regard. Her response was she would leave that until later to decide.

The next night in Fishers when we conducted our workshop, I related this conversation we had the night before (without giving any names), and the response of her ex-spouse was "Give me her name. Could I have her telephone number? I want to get a hold of her." :-)

Some people have a difficult time learning!

8

SESSION SIX — "WHAT DO I DO WITH ALL THAT MONEY I DON'T HAVE ANYMORE?"

The sixth session of our Divorce Recovery Workshop came with a different order.

After the Coffee and Informal Get-Together, the Show-And-Tell Time was eliminated because we brought in an Attorney to talk about the legal complications of divorce and it was felt the participants might be uncomfortable sharing some of their comments in the presence who was a stranger to these proceedings.

Before his appearance we had emphasized how important it is to employ separate attorneys rather than to try to save money by using the same attorney to represent both parties. Actually, the first attorney chosen to represent the divorcees is obligated by law to represent the first person asking for help.

The attorneys brought their own agenda dictated by their experience in representing divorcees. They talked about money (which can be scarce when plowing through divorce), child-custody issues, finding two houses in which to live, what to expect in court, pre-nuptual agreements, credit card debt, joint banking accounts, and about various other things that people may confront when settling this unhappy event.

We were fortunate to find attorneys who would not charge for their appearance at the Divorce Recovery Workshop presumably because there may have been individuals there that would need their help.

9

SESSION SEVEN — "TO LIVE AND LOVE AGAIN"

Six weeks ago when we first began this Divorce Recovery Workshop, had I begun with tonight's theme "TO LIVE AND LOVE AGAIN", I probably would have had my head lopped off by some of you (and deservedly so)! Some of you were struggling so hard with bitterness, anger, need for revenge, that the thought of loving again was clear out in left field somewhere, far out of your reach.

And now we are hearing some of you saying you would like to find a decent mate and know the joys of committed marriage. (As the old cigarette advertisement used to say), "You've come a long way, baby ... to get where you are today!" That is so thrilling for LaDonna and me to witness. It is so gratifying to see you reaching out to take a new hold on life again.

The two of us will never be able to adequately express our gratitude to each of you for giving us the high and holy privilege of walking down the private corridors of you minds and broken hearts to get to know you as the beautiful people you are. You have all proven yourself to be wonderful, beautiful, lovable people.

Some of you have already shared with us your anxieties, your joys, your successes in dating others since you have been in our workshop. If you people are merely normal (and we give you credit for being even a little bit above that), then nine chances out of ten you are going to date again. But more than that - you are going to marry again. 90% of divorced people marry again! Those are the current statistics.

I have a notion that many of you stopped dating even before your marriage was over. One of the beautiful things about my relationship with this wonderful lady is that we never stopped dating. It is still fun. We love to get out together and enjoy each other's company. We are still dating!

I can remember how exciting it was when we first started dating, and when we shared that first kiss. It literally sent cold chills up and down my back. (HER POPSICLE WAS DRIPPING.) :-)

It was probably scary for you back then ... not knowing if you would be accepted ... not knowing if you were making a mistake ... not knowing if he or she would be right for you. But that was one of the prices you had to pay. Jim Smoke tells us of a divorced man who shared this comment: "I resent being 37 years old and having to act, think and feel like a 17 year old again." Nevertheless, if your intention is to go on living and loving you will have to meet new friends, establish new relationships, and get back into the dating game again. That can be scary to some people. So about all a person can do is learn from the experiences

So let me talk first about the FEARS OF BUILDING NEW RELATIONSHIPS. Six major fears expressed most often in building new relationships with persons of the opposite sex are these:

1. CAN I BE SURE IT WILL LAST THIS NEXT TIME?

Sorry, but the honest answer to that question is "NO!" How many iron-clad guarantees does life offer? Not many, that is for sure. And marriage, particularly the second time around, carries with it no iron-clad guarantees. So about all a person can do is learn from the experiences of the past and walk hopefully, trustingly, and INTELLIGENTLY into the future ... with no guarantees ... but with a commitment to make it work next time around. We have tried since the first workshop session to help you determine what went wrong, to identify the garbage in your life, so that you won't take the same stuff into another relationship and doom it before it ever begins.

2. CAN I EVER TRUST ANOTHER MAN OR WOMAN?

I hope to God you can! You had better be able to trust again ... because you are cutting off approximately 50% of the friends God has made available to you if you never trust one of the opposite sex again. Not all men are bad. Not all women are bad. You can see that, can't you? Each of us deserves to be judged on our own individual merits. Let me remind you that you can't have deep meaningful friendships or relationships without developing deep trust levels. Trust is something that has to be earned. It grows with time. If you want to get from where you are now to where you want to be, trust has to be given a climate in which it can grow and prosper. You hurt most of all yourself when you throw your ability to trust out in the garbage can.

3. WILL I MAKE THE SAME MISTAKES ALL OVER AGAIN?

Maybe you will. I hope you don't. But you will if you haven't learned by your past mistakes and experiences. Most of us learn by trial and error. That is a costly and painful way to learn about marriage, but it does happen. Generally IT TAKES A PERSON BETWEEN ONE

AND TWO YEARS TO GAIN THE PROPER PER-
SPECTIVE ON DIVORCE AND LEARN THE
NEEDED LESSONS FROM THEIR MISTAKES. If
you don't learn from those mistakes and correct those
errors, you will take them into another relationship and
make those same mistakes all over again. Don't let that
happen to you.

4. CAN I BE HAPPY IF I MARRY AGAIN?

Not unless you are happy BEFORE you marry again.
Marriage does not give birth to happiness, and divorce
does not pronounce the benediction upon all possibili-
ties of knowing happiness again. Happiness begins deep
down inside of you. It is not dependent wholly upon out-
ward circumstances. Happiness is an attitude toward life.
And you can take this for what it is worth ... HAPPY
PEOPLE GENERALLY ATTRACT HAPPY PEOPLE.

5. WHAT IF I DON'T FIND ANYONE ELSE TO
MARRY?

Well that is a big "if". I'm not a gambling man, but I
would love to take a bet with you on whether or not you
will marry again. The odds are 9-1 in favor of remarriage.
Nine out of ten take the leap again.

Here is a strange one. Women keep asking us, "Where
are all the neat eligible men?" And the guys are asking,
"Where are all the really good women?" There are good
people everywhere. So keep yourself in circulation.
Don't go into hibernation. Get around to the good

places where good people gather. If you have a little bit of patience, a great lack of desperation, and a good measure of heart to look around a bit, you will find them out there.

I should say that not everyone will choose to remarry. Not everyone should. Only you can decide what is best for you. But chances are 9 out of 10 you are going to take the chance again.

6.   WILL I FEEL CONFIDENT AND SURE ENOUGH TO BEGIN DATING AGAIN?

It will probably be as scary for you after many years of married existence as it is for your sixteen year old son or daughter. But try to remember ... it may seem scary, but you can do it. You must do it ... if you are to live and love again.

Now I want to share some caution flags regarding the establishment of new relationships. These are Jim Smoke's ideas but they are my sentiments as well.

A.   HAVE YOU LEARNED ANYTHING ABOUT YOURSELF THROUGH YOUR DIVORCE?

Part of the growth process is learning who you really are. You ought not to think too seriously about dating (let alone remarriage) until you know something about your strengths and weaknesses that you did not know in your first marriage. There is a great risk that if in your first post-divorce dating relationship things do not lead to marriage, you may suffer the same devastating emotional shock upon the breakup of that relationship as you did with your divorce. It always hurts to learn that someone does not love you anymore. So keep cool and learn all there is to know about one of the most important persons in the world ... YOU! Don't allow yourself to become desperate.

B. HAS ENOUGH TIME ELAPSES TO LET THE DUST SETTLE?

The greatest mistake you can make is to remarry too quickly. Rebound marriages have a very poor track record, so give yourself time ... a year or two at the least.

C. ARE YOU BUILDING HEALTHY RELATIONSHIPS NOW?

A healthy relationship is not a totally dependent relationship where one person constantly drains the other. Each person has to offer the other something worthwhile in a healthy relationship. There has to be a balance between giving and receiving. A GOOD RULE IS TO DATE PEOPLE WHO ARE AT LAST AS FAR REMOVED FROM THEIR DIVORCE AS YOU ARE FROM YOURS.

D. HOW MUCH OF YOUR PAST ARE YOU DRAGGING WITH YOU INTO YOUR NEW RELATIONSHIP?

You can tell when you are gaining in your own growth and post-divorce adjustment when you talk less and less about your former failed marriage, your former spouse, your past divorce. If you spend your dating hours rehashing your divorce, you are dragging excess baggage along with you. If you don't get it behind you, you will make a poor risk for a good marriage partner.

All right — just in case I missed something — let's walk back over the past seven sessions and see where we have been.

1. Everybody hurts ... most hurt just like you when they go through divorce. We know how you feel. And we know what you feel. And whatever you feel, that is all right. Feelings come and go ... we can't help that. It is all right if the birds fly over your head, but you can't afford to let them make a nest in your hair. The best way you can deal with your hurts and feelings is to put a more positive interpretation on the events that trouble you. Take responsibility for your own feelings. No one else can make you feel what you do not choose to feel.

2. In order to get along with your ex-spouse, you have to deal with those feelings about your ex-spouse. Then those feelings give you a clue as to what went wrong in the relationship. The strongest feelings lead you to understand what kind of the seven divorces you suffered and alert you so that it will never happen to you again.

3. Forgiveness then is the turn-around point that will send you happily in another direction. Recognizing that you don't have to be perfect, admit your shortcomings to you ex-spouse, asking for their forgiveness and offering

your forgiveness to them as well. eclare that as far as you are concerned the war is over. And don't offer you ex any more ammunition to keep that war going.

4. Nobody else can take responsibility for yourself, your children, and your future. So step up to the plate and take your turn at bat. You have to do it for yourself. Nobody else can do it for you.

5. Accept your human sexuality as a beautiful gift from God. Don't spend it carelessly on someone who does not love you and commit himself or herself unreservedly to you. Sex can be beautiful only as you use it as God intended.

6. Financial considerations can crimp your style greatly in divorce. Take some financial wisdom that was offered you by the lawyer and put it to work so that this is one less thing to irritate you down the line. You can't take your money with you, as the old saying goes. (But did you ever try to go very far without it?)

7. Finally, take your time and do your homework before you commit yourself to another relationship. Don't be in a hurry. Don't be desperate. And don't make the same mistakes all over again. To live and love again is within each of your capacities. So get yourself ready ... and do it again ... this time with much more satisfying results than the first time (which was only practice for the real event).

10

THE BEGINNING AND THE END

We advertised rather extensively as we were getting ready to open our first Divorce Recovery Workshop. I received a telephone call one day from a fellow named Jim. He asked me to describe for him a little bit of what we were going to do in the workshop, our goals and plans and what we hoped to accomplish in it.

I was in the process of telling him the plans for the various sessions and he finally interrupted me by saying, "I don't know why I am even talking to you. The United Methodist Church has done nothing but cause me trouble since day one!" I said to him, "Jim, if that was designed to get my attention, it really worked. Now tell me, please, what you meant by that statement."

Jim told me he had what he thought was a pretty successful life and a pretty successful marriage. Then he came home from work early one afternoon to find his wife and his United Methodist Church minister in bed with each other. He said, "That preacher got my wife, my house, and got half of my net worth. He ruined my life. That is why I don't know why I am even talking to you about a Divorce Recovery Workshop. I just don't know if such a workshop would work for me."

I expressed my sincere apology for what had happened to him and then I suggested he come for a session or two with no obligation to pay or stay. If he found some benefit in it he could continue. Otherwise he could walk away and that would be the end of that.

Jim came. He got into the program quite determinedly and stayed to the very end. When that first Divorce Recovery Workshop was over, he came to me wanting to know if he could come to our Sunday Worship Service to say "Thanks" for the experience he had there. I said, "Jim, the service is already planned quite tight, and I can only afford to give you two ... maybe three minutes ... to speak." He agreed and the next Sunday morning he was there early on the front row ready to go.

Since this was the first Divorce Recovery Workshop our church had ever conducted, many in our congregation had no idea what we were doing there or why we were doing it. There was even a question among some if we should be doing a program such as this.

I introduced Jim as one of the participants in the DRW and he came to the pulpit and opened up his heart to the waiting congregation. He told them of our first telephone conversation together and how the United Methodist Church had brought tragedy to his life through the betrayal of his trust in his minister. The people were astonished as he related to them how this former United Methodist Church minister stole his wife, his home, and half of his monetary worth.

He reiterated how the United Methodist Church had taken the very life out of him. And then he said, "I am here this morning to thank this church for giving me a new lease on life. I will ever be grateful to you because you have put new life where there was once dead meaning and purpose."

There was not a dry eye in the congregation when he finished his speech that morning.. The sermon that followed (whatever it was) really wasn't necessary after he had concluded his expression of thanks. And whatever elements of doubt about the necessity of that new program vanquished in the instant he sat down again with the audience clapping loudly even through their tears.

11

SERMON ON DIVORCE

"WHAT YOU SHOULD KNOW ABOUT DIVORCE ... "
(I Corinthians 7:10-17)

Sermon preached by Rev. Nelson M. Chamberlin
Fishers United Methodist Church   (8/23/1981)

The most dangerous thing the Christian Church has to offer this world is a person who glibly quotes Scripture without knowing what the Scripture is saying.

We have given many of that sort to the world, unfortunately. Until a person knows WHO is doing the talking (or writing); and until one knows TO WHOM this was written or spoken; and until one knows WHY this was written; and until one knows WHAT IT MEANT to its intended recipients in their day ... one cannot apply these Scriptures to our day and to our lives without genuine understanding.

It is absolutely essential for us to know the context of the Holy Scripture when we quote it and when we talk to others about it. To do less than that is to do violence to the Scripture and to do harm to people who deserve no such treatment.

We have done harm to people when we have talked unadvisedly about divorce. There are basically three sections of Scripture that deal with "divorce." There is (1) the Old Testament section in Deuteronomy 24:1-4 in which Moses talks about the PERMISSIBLE PRACTICE (or the permissible ideal) of his day. In the Old Testament days people were justified (they thought) by the keeping of the Law, and Moses was saying, "Yes, the ideal — the perfect — will of God is that when people pledge their love and loyalty and faith to one another they will then live together for the rest of their natural lives. But in case you cannot do that, here are certain exceptions allowable to that rule ... you may get a divorce for the following reasons ... "

Now to quote the Old Testament Scriptures from Deuteronomy 24, you have to realize that this was written by a man to a people who were living under the Old Testament Law, who sought to be justified by the keeping of that Law, and therefore this passage does not apply to us in the same way it applied to them.

Centuries later Jesus said, "That was given because of the hardness of their hearts." It was all right then because those people were trying to justify themselves by the keeping of the Law, but they could not do it for themselves. So God made certain exceptions.

Next we come to (2) the New Testament, particularly to Matthew 19:3-9; (the Sermon on the Mount ... Matthew 5:31-32); Mark 10:11-12 and Luke 16:18. In these passages Jesus is saying in essence, "My friends, there is only one real reason in God's Kingdom for dissolving a marriage. A marriage is dead only ... ONLY when there has been adultery or fornication complicating the relationship."

It is essential to realize that when you quote those prohibitions against divorce that Jesus was talking about the Coming Kingdom. He was offering that Kingdom to the people but they promptly rejected it. So that Kingdom was not established in its fullness then. It is not established in its fullness even in this day. It will not be established in its fullness until that day when Jesus Christ comes back to earth to rule and reign. And He will rule then with an iron hand. No evil will be allowed. No wrong will be tolerated. In that day the perfect ideal of marriage (which Jesus expresses here) will be fulfilled.

It is very important for us to realize when we read Jesus' words in the Gospels (particularly these words) that He is talking about a PERFECT IDEAL that will be established in The Kingdom Age. If you are tempted to literally apply all of these principles and ideals to the present age and make them totally obligatory upon us, then you must remember some of the same words Jesus said in that Kingdom Literature. "Unless your righteousness exceeds the righteousness of the Scribes and Pharisees, you don't have chance." (Do you give multiple tithes of your income as they did? Do you worship as regularly and faithfully as they did? Are you as devoted to the Law as they were?) Jesus described their righteousness and it far exceeds ours outwardly.

Jesus went on to say, "Be ye therefore perfect, even as your Father in Heaven is perfect." I haven't met anyone yet who measures up to that PERFECT IDEAL yet. Have you? Someday when His Kingdom shall be fully established ... but not yet! We are not perfect, and we are not righteous in ourselves. So when we look at Jesus' PERFECT IDEAL for marriage, we have to remember that this is Kingdom Literature. It is a perfect ideal toward which God wants us to strive, and yet it is not an ideal to which all people can measure up.

Now we move the (3) a third section of the Holy Scriptures which comes to us in the Epistle of Paul to the Corinthians (I Corinthians 7:10-17). This passage of Scripture is written to the people of Corinth. Corinth was a wicked, wicked little town in Greece. It was renowned for its wickedness! Divorce was a very easy thing there in that day ... way too easy! All a man had to do was to say, "I want a divorce" and that was it!

He did not even have to offer a reason for divorce. It was automatically granted to him on request. And if a woman chose to be divorced, she only had to offer some specific reason and she too would be granted her request. So the Corinthian Christians wrote to St. Paul and asked him, "Hey! What shall we do with this matter of marriage and divorce in our society?" Paul responded with these words:

"To the married I give charge, not I but the Lord, that the wife should not separate from her husband (B-U-T if she does, let her remain single or else be reconciled to her husband) — and that the husband should not divorce his wife.

"To the rest I say, not the Lord, that if any brother has a wife who is an unbeliever, and she consents to live with him, he should not divorce her. If any woman has a husband who is an unbeliever, and he consents to live with her, she should not divorce him. For the unbelieving wife is consecrated through her husband. Otherwise you children would be unclean, but as it is they are holy.

"B-U-T if the unbelieving partner desires to separate (and that word means "DIVORCE" ... there is no such formality in the ancient Corinthian society as separation as we know it today ... you were married or you were divorced), let it be so; in such a case the brother or sister is not bound (the word here is "SLAVE") to that relationship, FOR GOD HAS CALLED US TO PEACE.

Wife, how do you know whether you will save your husband? Husband, how do you know whether you will save your wife?

"Only, let everyone lead the life which the Lord has assigned to him, and in which God has called him. This is my rule in all the churches."

Paul wrote to the Corinthians on that occasion about the great stress that was about to come upon them. The great stress that came upon the Corinthians was that the Romans reached out in their persecution, and the Jews as well, and tried to run them into the ground and destroy them as an unworthy cult. Paul realized that in the coming days of persecution it might be necessary for some people either to deny their faith, or to sacrifice their children to those cruel Romans. So he said, "If you have a husband or wife who does not believe the way you do, and if they want out of the relationship because of that stress, it is O.K. You are not bound."

Jesus did not say that (of course), but Paul did. And Paul was not contradicting Jesus when he wrote this because Paul was speaking from a different platform and different circumstances that Jesus. Jesus spoke from the platform of THE IDEAL KINGDOM which is yet to be established — THE PERFECT AND IDEAL KINGDOM in which no wrong will be tolerated. St. Paul wrote from the stage of Corinth where God's grace and love and forgiveness were operative. God was saying through Paul, "You are not there yet, people. You are not yet perfected. But I will not hold that against you so long as your faith is in Me through Jesus Christ. I will account that to you as righteousness, and I will forgive you when you do wrong."

So Moses spoke about THE PERMISSIBLE IDEAL of marriage and divorce. Jesus spoke about THE PERFECT IDEAL of marriage and divorce. And Paul spoke about THE PRACTICAL IDEAL of marriage and divorce.

We are less than perfect human beings. So God makes provision for those who are less than perfect. Paul said that marriage was made for people and people are not necessarily made for marriage. The key to this (I think) was Paul's insistence that THERE NEEDS TO BE PEACE. "For this we were created," he said "that we might have peace." He was talking about peace with God … yes, but he was also talking about our peace with one another in our marital relationships. So Paul said there are going to be occasions when it might become necessary to divorce rather than to stay together and be slain by staying in that relationship.

Now — why all the difficult passages? Why all the prohibitions? Why these different IDEALS expressed in the Holy Scriptures regarding marriage and its permanence? It is because God knew from the beginning of the foundations of the earth what when we say "Yes" to each

other — "I will love you forever" — and then go back on
that promise there is going to be deep hurt involved.
And God is saying, 'I DON'T WANT YOU TO GET
HURT! I DON'T WANT THIS TO HAPPEN TO
YOU. I WISH FOR YOU TO BE COMMITTED SO
FULLY TO EACH OTHER THAT YOU WILL
NEVER EXPERIENCE THIS DEVASTATING HURT
THAT GOES WITH DIVORCE."

But St. Paul comes along to add, "IF YOU ARE
EXPERIENCING HURT, AND YOU ARE JUST
SLAYING EACH OTHER WITH WORDS OR
ACTIONS ... MAYBE IT IS BETTER TO GET OUT
THAN TO KEEP KILLING EACH OTHER
STAYING TOGETHER."

I can testify that it really hurts when people hear
somebody else say, "I loved you, but I don't love you
anymore." On any given Sunday I can look out past this
pulpit and see numerous people who, were it not for the
fact that this church has reached out to them and said,
"We love you and we care about you," those persons
would be dead right now. They have been hurt so badly
by someone denying them love that they would almost
have wanted to die.

In our Divorce Recovery Workshops about 50% of the
participants will tell us they were suicidal at one point in
their lives. Another 40% don't come right out and say it
in so many words, but we catch it anyway! What I am

trying to tell you, my friends, is that when somebody says "I don't love you anymore" it hurts ... and God says, "I DON'T WANT YOU TO HURT LIKE THAT!" It hurts almost to the point of death.

The sad truth of the matter however is that the Christian Church for many years has taken the Old Testament position where we sit in judgment of those people who have not been able to live up to the high demands of God's Law. But that is not where you and I are coming from in this day. We are coming not from a position of judgment and punishment, but from the arena of God's Love and Grace and Forgiveness. Need I remind you THERE IS NO SIN (NOT EVEN DIVORCE) THAT IS SO GREAT HE IS UNWILLING TO FORGIVE IT!

If a person commits murder, we say "That's all right! We can forgive you." If a person commits thievery, we say "We can forgive that!" If a person lies, we say "No problem. I can forgive that." But the unfortunate attitude of the Church too often has been, "BUT IF YOU ARE DIVORCED, THERE IS NO FORGIVENESS FOR YOU. THAT IS ONE SIN THAT GOD CANNOT FORGIVE (AND NEITHER CAN WE)!"

Hogwash! There is nothing further from the truth than that. The only sin that God cannot forgive is that sin where we keep pushing Him away until He is so far away we cannot hear His voice anymore. And the inability of God to forgive us in that instance is not because God lacks the power or desire to forgive. It is because we lack the receptivity to accept His forgiveness. We cannot hear His voice anymore.

There is no sin too great for God to be able to forgive. God's IDEAL (and it is a good one) is that we should never say "I love you" and then back up on that promise because there is just so much hurt involved in a thing like that when it happens. But even if we err at that point (as in many other points as well), He wants to forgive us. 41% of first-time marriages are going down the drain today. The current estimate is that 50% of all the marriages that are being performed today will end up in the divorce courts. 59% of second marriages are doomed to fail. 83% of third marriages are not going to make it.

Have you heard enough? It is not that second or third marriages cannot work. It is that often people do not work through the problems of their first marriage, and they bring the same garbage into the second and third and fourth marriage they brought into the first — and they go through the same hurt all over again.

Here is God today saying to His children, "Here is MY IDEAL. I lay it out for you to strive after. If you strive for it and achieve it, you will save yourself untold grief, sorrow and hurt in a world that is too full of hurt already. But if you are not able to achieve this ideal, then I understand your weakness. I still love. I still care. I still forgive."

Now here comes the crux of this whole matter. It seems to me that the task of the Church today is not to look down our noses upon those who have had unhappy relationships and who have not been able to keep them together and who have gone through divorce. Rather our task as caring Christians should be to look upon these individuals who have gone through the heartbreak and trauma of divorce and say, "We still love you. We still care about you, friend. We want to identify with you in your grief."

Unfortunately that has not always been the testimony of the Church. But increasingly it is the testimony of this congregation. We offer Divorce Recovery Workshops continually to help these sufferers cope with their hurt. Basically the premise is this: EVEN AS GOD LOVES US AND FORGIVES US IN ALL OUR WEAKNESS, WE ARE AMBASSADORS OF CHRIST. WE ARE AGENTS OF RECONCILIATION TO THOSE WHO ARE HURTING BADLY. WE OFFER TO THEM IN THE NAME OF JESUS CHRIST OUR LOVE AND UNDERSTANDING AND ACCEPTANCE BECAUSE THOSE WHO GO THROUGH THE HEARTBREAK OF DIVORCE ARE PEOPLE WHO HURT LIKE NOBODY SHOULD EVER HAVE TO HURT.

May God help each of us to look not in a judgmental way but in a loving way toward those who have not been able to achieve the perfect ideal of marriage. And may God help each of us to focus on that Ideal of an Enduring Marriage so that we and others about us will not have to suffer the hurt that comes when someone says, "I don't love you anymore."

Let us pray.

O Lord, if we have been less than understanding — If we have been less than caring — If we have been less than faithful to Your WHOLE TRUTH, forgive us. And for all of those who are experiencing rocky, difficult times in their marital relationships right now, O God give them the courage to communicate, to trust, and to love and work out those problems. And if there are those who cannot do this, help them to know that they are still loveable, that they are still good, that they are still accepted by You even though sometimes their actions fall far short of Your Perfect Ideal.

Now Lord, as we make our way from this place today, may we go with renewed and vigorous determination to live according to Your ideal for us. But may we also go with the assurance that when we are weak and when we fail, You are still there to lift us up and help us go on. May we, with the same comfort by which we have been comforted, reach out to comfort those who are in deepest pain.

Through our Lord Jesus Christ, we pray. Amen.

people do not work through

of all marriages that are being performed today will
end up in the divorce courts in the future.

12

ADDENDUMS

GUIDELINES FOR SUCCESSFUL SINGLE PARENTING
(by Jim Smoke)

1. Don't try to be both parents to your children.
2. Don't force your children into playing the role of the departed parent.
3. Be the parent you are. Don't abdicate your parent position for that of a big brother, big sister, friend, buddy or pal.
4. Be honest with your children. Tell the truth about what is going on.
5. Don't put your ex-spouse down in front of your children.
6. Don't make your children undercover agents who report on the other parent's activities.

7. The children of divorce need both a mother and a father. Don't deny them this right because of your anger, hostility, guilt or vengeance.

8. Don't become a "Disneyland Daddy" or a "Magic Mountain Momma".

9. Share your dating life and social interest with your children.

10. Help your children keep the good memories of your past marriage alive.

11. Work out a management and existence structure for your children with your ex-spouse.

12. If possible, try not to disrupt the many areas in your children's lives that offer them safety and security.

13. If your child does not resume normal development and growth in his life within a year of the divorce, he may need the special care and help of a professional counselor.

LETTING GO

❋ To let go doesn't mean to stop caring, it means I can't do it for someone else.

❋ To let go is not to cut myself off, it's the realization that I don't control another.

❋ To let go is not to enable, but to allow learning from natural consequences.

❋ To let go is to admit powerlessness, which means the outcome is not in my hands.

❋ To let go is not to try to change or blame another, I can only change myself.

❋ To let go is not to care for, but to care about.

❋ To let go is not to fix, but to be supportive.

❋ To let go is not to judge, but to allow another to be a human being.

❋ To let go is not to be in the middle arranging all the outcomes, but to allow others to affect their own outcomes.

❋ To let go is not to be protective, it is to permit another to face reality.

❋ To let go is not to deny but to accept.

❋ To let go is not to nag, scold, or argue, but to search out my own shortcomings and to correct them.

❋ To let go is not to adjust everything to my desires but to take each day as it comes and to cherish the moment.

❋ To let go is not to criticize and regulate anyone but to try to become what I dream I can be.

❋ To let go is not to regret the past but to grow and live for the future.

❋ To let go is to fear less and love more.

— Author Unknown

ATTITUDE (BY CHARLES SWINDOLL)

"The longer I live, the more I realize the impact of attitude on life. Attitude, to me, is more important than facts. It is more important than the past, than education, than money, than circumstances, than failures, than successes, than what other people think or say or do. It is more important than appearance, giftedness or skill. It will make or break a company ... a church ... a home."

"The remarkable thing is that we have a choice every day regarding the attitude we will embrace for that day. We cannot change our past ... we cannot change the fact that people will act in a certain way. We cannot change the inevitable. The only thing we can do is play on the one string we have, and that is our attitude ... I am convcinced that life is 10 percent what happens to me and 90 percent how I react to it. And so iut is with you ... we are in charge of our Attitudes!"

AUTOBIOGRAPHY IN FIVE SHORT CHAPTERS
(BY PORTIA NELSON)
I.
I walk down the street.
>   There is a deep hole in the sidewalk.
>   I fall in.
>   I am lost ... I am helpless.
>   It isn't my fault.
>   It takes forever to get out.
II.
I walk down the same street.
>   There is a deep hole in the sidewalk.
>   I pretend I don't see it.
>   I fall in again.

I can't believe I am in the same place,
But it isn't my fault.

III.

I walk down the same street.
There is a deep hole in the sidewalk.
I see it there.
I still fall in ... it's a habit,
my eyes are open.
I know where I am.
It is my fault.
I get out immediately.

IV.

I walk down the same street.
There is a deep hole in the sidewalk.
I walk around it.

V.

I walk down another street.

GUIDELINES FOR SINGLE PARENTING
GUIDELINES FOR SUCCESSFUL SINGLE PARENTING
(by Jim Smoke)

1. Don't try to be both parents to your children.

2. Don't force your children into playing the role of the departed parent.

3. Be the parent you are. Don't abdicate your parent position for that of a big brother, big sister, friend, buddy or pal.

4. Be honest with your children. Tell the truth about what is going on.

5. Don't put your ex-spouse down in front of your children.

6. Don't make your children undercover agents who report on the other parent's activities.

7. The children of divorce need both a mother and a father. Don't deny them this right because of your anger, hostility, guilt or vengeance.

8. Don't become a "Disneyland Daddy" or a "Magic Mountain Momma".

9. Share your dating life and social interest with your children.

10. Help your children keep the good memories of your past marriage alive.

11. Work out a management and existence structure for your children with your ex-spouse.

12. If possible, try not to disrupt the many areas in your children's lives that offer them safety and security.

13. If your child does not resume normal development and growth in his life within a year of the divorce, he may need the special care and help of a professional counselor.

FORGIVENESS

Forgiveness is the bud's fragrance under the boot hell that crushed it.

Dear Abby: I love reading your column. A couple of years ago I read a piece on forgiveness and realized that, like many other people, I don't know how to forgive or ask for forgiveness. You column helped. Would you please run it again?

Mrs. G.S.K.P., Lake Worth, Fla.

Dear Mrs. G.S.P.K.: Pleased to oblige. Since this is International Forgiveness Week, your letter is timely. The poem you requested was written by George Roemisch.

FORGIVENESS

Forgiveness is the wind-blown bud
Which blooms in placid beauty at Verdun.

Forgiveness is the tiny slate-gray sparrow
Which has built its nest of twigs and string
Among the shards of glass upon the wall of shame.

Forgiveness is the child who laughs in merry ecstasy
Beneath the toothed fence that closes in Da Nang.

Forgiveness is the fragrance of the violet
Which still clings fast to the heel that crushed it.

Forgiveness is the broken dream
Which hides itself within the corner of the mind
Oft called forgetfulness so that it will not bring
Pain to the dreamer.

Forgiveness is the reed
Which stands up straight and green

When nature's mighty rampage halts, full spent.
Forgiveness is a God who will not leave us
After all we've done.

So, dear readers, a gentle reminder: If perchance you are the "heel" that crushed the violet — this is the week to seek forgiveness.

QUOTES ON FORGIVENESS

Trying to "get even" becomes a moral boomerang that does more harm to us than to our enemies.

A strong feeling of resentment is just as likely to cause disease as is a germ. Many people could improve their health by washing their hearts clean of ill-will and resentment.

An "unforgiving" persons is an "unforgiven" person.

A grudge is too heavy a load for anyone to carry.

COMES THE DAWN
After a while you learn the subtle difference
Between holding a hand and chaining a soul,
And you learn that love doesn't mean leaning
And company doesn't mean security,
And you begin to understand that kisses aren't contracts,
And presents are promises,
And you begin to accept your defeats
With your head held high and your eyes open,
With the grace of a woman, not the grief of a child.

You learn to build your roads
On today because tomorrow's ground
Is too uncertain for plans, and futures have
A way of falling down in mid-flight.
After a while you learn that even sunshine
Burns if you get too much,
So you plant your own garden and decorate
Your own soul, instead of waiting
For someone to bring you flowers.
And you learn that you really can endure,
That you really have worth,
And learn and learn ... and you learn
With every good-bye you learn.

THE RULES OF ROMANCE (KNIGHT RIDDER NEWSPAPERS)

* **Abandon the passion delusion:** Passion declines over time. This is natural and normal, not horrible.
* **Romantic feelings can't be forced:** You can't talk yourself into falling in love. Nor can you engineer situations to stir passion you don't feel.
* **Relationships are hard work:** You must instantly put effort into maintaining a relationship, just as you would a career, or a car.

THERE ARE MANY NONBAR PLACES TO MEET SINGLES

Is the singles bar the only place to meet a potential date? Where else can you go? What else can you do?

Some answers from Nina Atwood, a licensed therapist and Relationship coach, who asked participants in one of her workshops about meeting places.

Home:

* Play an instrument on your front porch/patio/front yard
* Hang out at your neighborhood or apartment pool
* Attend Crimewatch meetings
* Do yard work and talk to passersby
* Introduce yourself to neighbors.

Work:

* Volunteer groups
* Social groups or happy hours after work
* Introduce yourself to one person outside your immediate work group each day
* Talk to riders on elevators
* Hang around the copier/coffee machine/break room

Shopping:

* At the grocery store, ask for advice on certain foods
* Hang out in bookstore coffee shops

Religious:

* Attend a church or synagogue
* Join a singles Sunday School Class

Recreation:

❋ Join special interest groups

❋ Attend sporting events, concerts, and plays and mingle during breaks

❋ Attend festivals, street fairs and flea markets

Education:

❋ Take adult education classes

❋ Check into offerings at public libraries

UNHAPPY ENDINGS IF COUPLES CO-HABIT (BY MAGGIE GALLAGHER - UNIVERSAL PRESS SYNDICATE)

Valentine's day has arrived and the University of Michigan's Professor Pamela Smock has released an impressive report on co-habituation just in the nick of time.

Dear Professor Smock:

The good news is, I just heard your study reported on the top-rated *Z100 Z-Morning Zoo*. The bad news is, they mistakenly reported that 50 percent of households are now co-habiting. Things are not that bad. But the '90s was definitely the decade for living together.

Since just the late '80s, the proportion of women in their late 30s who have ever co-habited jumped from 30 percent to 48 percent. Many of these co-habiting couples have children in the household, most often the child of just one partner.

But about 40 percent of unwed births are now to co-habiting couples — 50 percent of white and Latino women and about a quarter of black women. Most of the increase in out-of-wedlock births in the '90s is due to increased births to co-habiting two-parent families, and not to lone women. More couples driven in part by divorce anxiety, are deciding they can make families without the formality of legal, public vow.

Don't last long

Unfortunately for the babies, these fragile, informal families mostly do not last long. "Only about one-sixth of co-habitations last at least three years, and only a 10th last five years or more," notes Smock.

By contrast, at current divorce rates, almost six out of ten couples who marry for the first time created a bond that will last until the death of one partner. When it comes to creating a tie between lovers so firm a child's heart can rely upon it, we haven't invented anything that tops the marriage vow.

But what about the 55 percent of co-habitations that end in marriage? Isn't living together first a good investment? The answer, in a word, is no. Married couples who co-habited first have more relationship problems and divorces than couples who wait to say "I do" before moving in together. Living together first definitely won't help you make a happy marriage, and it may hurt.

Sorry, it seems that women who live with men end up doing almost as much housework as wives. But their male partners don't share their income, accept responsibility for bread-winning, or promise to support them if the going gets tough, or even be there for the baby. For women, the co-habiting rule seems to be most all the work and none of the protection of marriage.

Worse off than if married

As Professor Smock concludes: "Given evidence that co-habiting couples are less likely to pool income than married couples (Blumstein & Schwartz, 1983), the find of these housework studies imply that co-habiting women are — in a very important sense — worse off than married women."

In these peculiar days, when otherwise intelligent women take getting your boyfriend to move in and mooch off your labor and love without commitment as a sign of deepening affection, the entire canon of love poetry needs revising.

How do I love thee? Let me count the ways.

I love thee to the depth and breadth my soul can reach.

While scrubbing your dishes, and washing your floors:

And having your babies, while you claim your freedom;

Your leisure, your paycheck and my labor as you own.

Not much, I know. But this I's afraid — so afraid — is perhaps as it gets.

Happy Valentine's Day 2000

PRAYER FOR THE DIVORCED (author unknown)
God, Master of Union and Disunion,
Teach me how I may now walk
Alone and strong.
Heal my wounds;
Let the scar tissue of Thy bounty
Cover these bruises and hurts
That I may again be a single person
Adjusted to new days.
Grant me a heart of wisdom,
Make me know the laughter which is nolt giddy,
The affection which is not frightened.
Keep far from me thoughts of evil and despair.
May I realize that the past chapter of my life
Is closed and will not open again.
The anticipated theme of my life has changed,
The expected story end will not come.
Shall I moan at the turn of the plot?
Rather, remembering without anger's thrust,
Recalling without repetitive pain of regret,
Teach me again to write and read
That I may convert this unexpected epilogue
Into a new preface and a new poem.
Muddled gloom over,
Tension days passed,

Let bitterness of thought fade,
Harshness of memory attenuate,
Make me move on in love and kindness.

CPSIA information can be obtained at www.ICGtesting.com
Printed in the USA
LVOW131427210613

339726LV00002B/6/P